Cherished
Baby and Child

A practical guide for parents on the most common conditions that can affect your baby and child.
And the solutions...

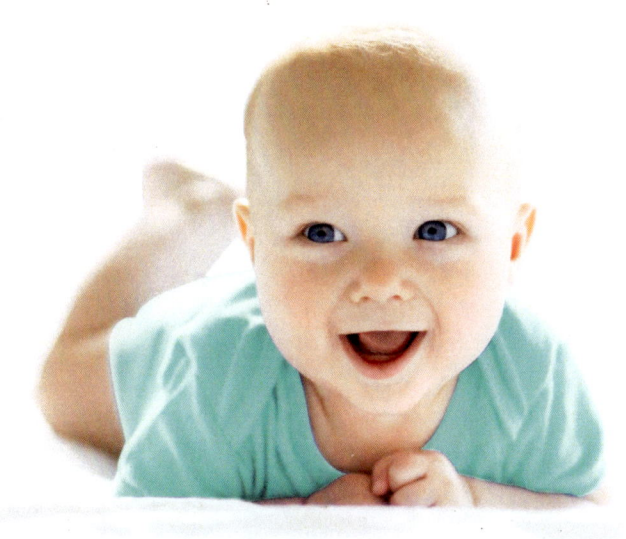

Frank Kelleher, *Paediatric Osteopath* D.O., R.N.M.H., G.Os.C., M.O.C.I.

and

Rose Kelleher, *Midwife* R.G.N., R.M.

Cherished Baby and Child © 2019 by Frank & Rose Kelleher. All rights reserved.

No part of this book may be reproduced in any form or by any electronic or mechanical means including information storage and retrieval systems, without permission in writing from the author. The only exception is by a reviewer, who may quote short excerpts in a review.

This book is not intended as a substitute for medical diagnosis, treatment or advice from a qualified health professional. You should use the information at your own risk. Note that most of the information contained in this book is based on the authors' personal experience of treating babies and children over the last twenty years. Though the authors have made every reasonable attempt to ensure accuracy of the contents, they assume no responsibility for errors or omissions. No gratuity or commercial benefit has been received for the reference to any product, service or company, organisation or website.

Photographs courtesy of shutterstock.com

Designed and Printed by Lettertec.

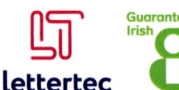

*This book is dedicated to our four
amazing children –
Niall, Lauren, Livy and Gavin.*

cherished
[cher-ish-ed]
to hold or treat as dear; feel love for:
to cherish one's native land.

to care for tenderly; nurture:
to cherish a child.

About the Authors

Frank Kelleher D.O., R.N.M.H., G.Os.C., M.O.C.I.

Frank has been working in healthcare for more than 30 years. He began his People with Learning Disability (PLD) training at Cope Foundation, Cork in 1987 and continued to work in this area in London where he was the Director of PLD Nursing Services for the Richmond, Twickenham and Roehampton Healthcare Trust. His osteopathy journey began in London in 1992. He trained at the London School of Osteopathy and qualified in 1997. He returned to Cork in 1998 with Rose and their children and set up his own clinic. Since then he has specialised in paediatric care and has built up a very busy practice. He has a far-reaching reputation, with parents travelling from all over Ireland to see him. One of Frank's main objectives is to give parents as much information as possible about their child's health. He is passionate about giving parents an effective plan to help them manage and resolve the condition affecting their little one.

Rose Kelleher R.G.N., R.M.

Rose is a General Nurse and a Midwife. She has worked in London as a Midwife and was a Practice Nurse in a GP Surgery in Richmond, Surrey. On returning to Cork in 1998, she started working with Frank and over the last twenty years has helped Frank to build up the business to where it is now. Having a mum of four, a nurse and a midwife managing the clinic has been a huge advantage over the years. Rose has a genuine empathy for the mums we see in the clinic and can often offer them the advice her many years of experience have given her.

Contents

Introduction	1
Delivery and its effects on baby	5
The early weeks	11
Infant reflux	15
Lactose overload	37
Colic and Gut Health	51
Cow's Milk Protein Allergy	59
Sleep	73
Tongue-tie	85
Plagiocephaly	93
Ear infections and glue ear	103
Behaviour, anxiety and concentration	113
Night terrors	121
Down's syndrome	127
Constipation	133
Symptom management chart	143
Notes	150

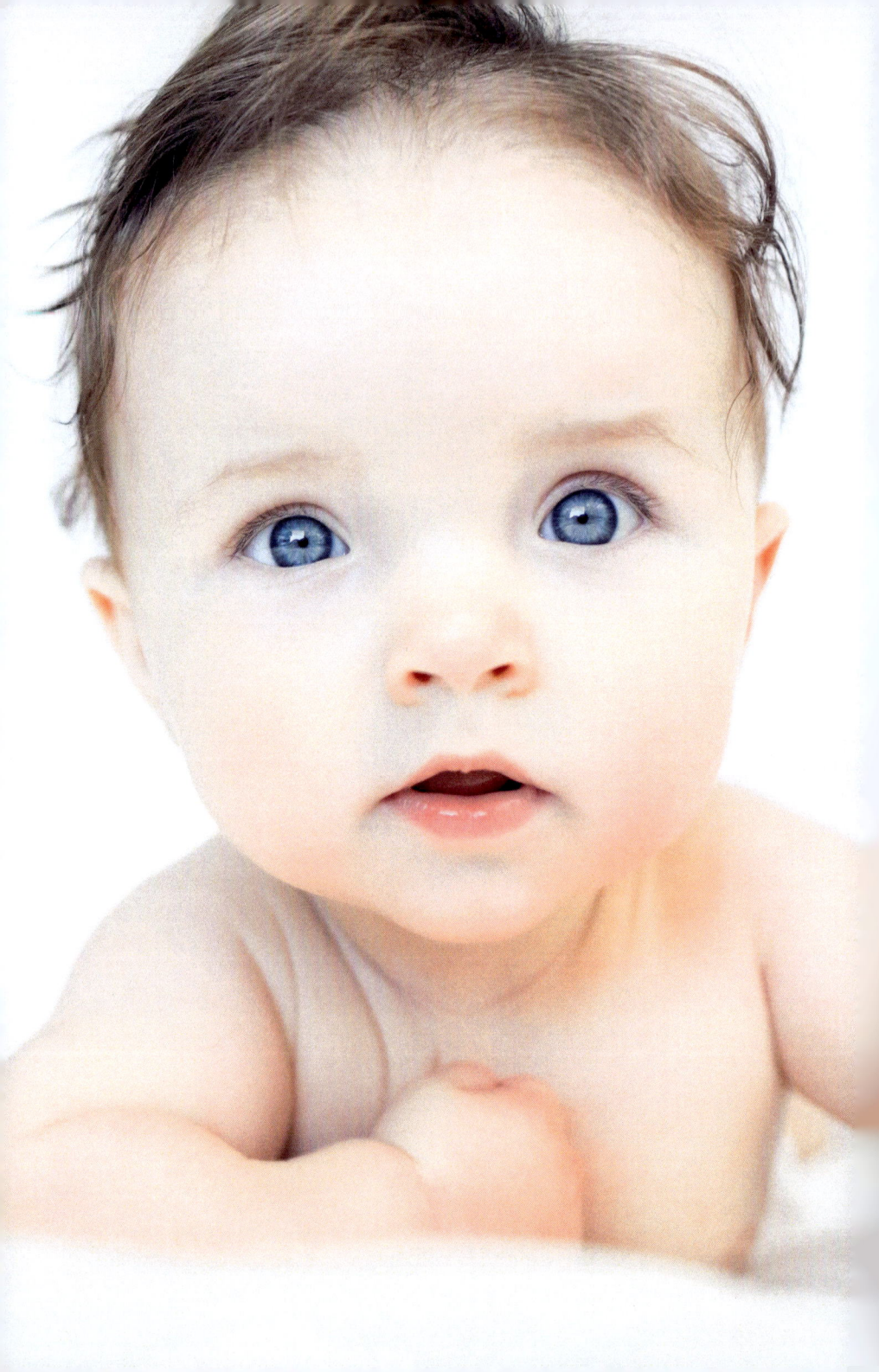

Introduction

This book has been a long-time dream for us. We have both worked in healthcare for over 30 years—Frank started out in disability nursing before moving on to osteopathy, and Rose was a nurse and a midwife. We have been working with babies and children for almost twenty years, having seen more than 10,000 babies during this time. Over the years we have treated many of the most common issues that can cause distress for little ones.

We have been determined to find the best solutions for these issues and have always valued the importance of explaining what's happening in simple terms to parents. We know only too well how upsetting it is to be the parent of a small baby or child, who is in obvious distress, and not know what to do to make things better (or even worse, to have your concerns dismissed because you are a "first time Mum").

Our first son was born soon after we moved to London. We know now that he had reflux, but our doctor never diagnosed his condition and we very often felt lost. We understand how it is to feel helpless as the parents of a small distressed baby. Once parents understand why their little one is upset and unsettled, and what they can do to help, it allows them to cope with it better. We love to give parents a plan and some reassurance that all is well. First-time parents can feel especially vulnerable when things don't go right. They have so many questions and often think that no-one is listening to them. We have always listened to what parents say about their baby as they are the people who know their baby best. *Cherished Baby and Child* looks at the most common conditions we have seen at our clinic over the last twenty years, and, for each, provides a detailed description of the condition itself and the solutions that have worked for the babies and children we have seen.

Our little ones have all received cranial osteopathic treatment along with the advice we have given to parents, and in these cases, this treatment will also have had a very beneficial effect on the presenting condition. In each chapter we have explained how cranial osteopathy helps, to allow you to decide if you wish to take your child to a

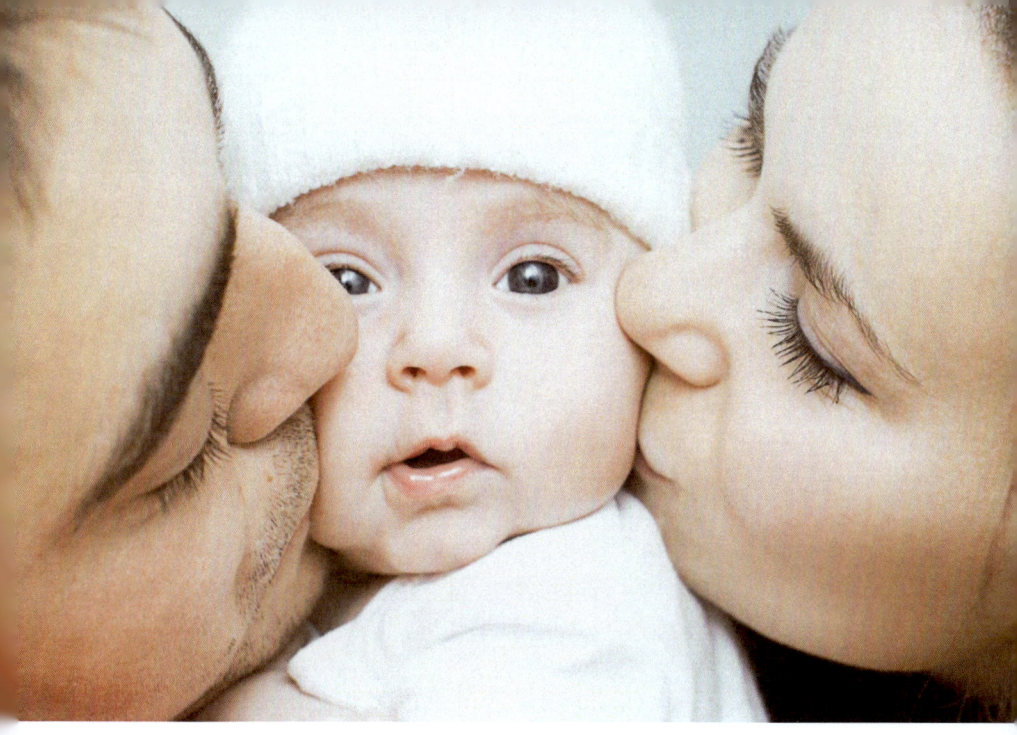

paediatric osteopath in addition to the advice the book offers. Some conditions will benefit more from cranial osteopathy than others, but the treatment will be suitable for all the conditions mentioned in the book.

We start the book where your journey starts, the birth of your baby. Some factors involved in the delivery can have an effect on baby and it's best to be aware of this and seek assistance if needed early. We have seen babies only days old where there has been a difficult delivery and parents want treatment sooner rather than later. The fourth trimester is then discussed as this is a time when baby needs so much of your attention. It's a wonderful few weeks to bond with and get to know your little one.

Most of the babies we see at our clinic come for treatment for a digestive disorder. The next few chapters look at the different digestive issues we see every day. Some of the conditions we discuss can be complicated to treat and, in these cases, you will need the advice of your medical practitioner. Remember that every child is different and while we have done our best to explain the conditions and the treatment options in as much detail as possible, it is always wise to have your child reviewed by a medical practitioner who can assess them fully and offer their expertise. No book can replace a face-to-face examination and assessment by the right practitioner.

As children get older the reasons why we see them change. Sleep, congestion, ear infections and glue ear are common. We see children up to early teenage years, but it is babies and toddlers who mostly fill our day.

We are very fortunate to work in paediatrics. We remind ourselves of this very often and can honestly say that we love our job. Every child we see is special to us. This book is an opportunity for us to change the lives of so many more families by giving parents the information they need to help their baby. We genuinely hope that *Cherished Baby and Child* will offer you a successful solution to your concerns about your little one. As parents of four wonderful children ourselves, we only want to help others to enjoy those magical years by giving you our solutions to some of the frequently occurring conditions that can disrupt your little cherished one's life.

Frank and Rose

Delivery and its effects on baby

The day a baby is born is an amazing, life-changing event. For most mums and babies, birth itself will be straightforward and without any complications. While first babies can take a little longer, second and subsequent babies are generally a little faster in arriving. Mums and babies are designed for a normal delivery and in the vast majority of cases, that's exactly what happens. For other mums and babies however, it can be a very different experience. While a long or difficult labour and/or delivery does not necessarily mean that baby will need a little assistance afterwards, it may increase the probability of baby having some of the conditions we see at our clinic.

There are a few things that can cause distress for your little one as they enter the world. The obvious one is the type of delivery baby has. Some deliveries are more difficult than others but the types of deliveries that seem to cause most difficulty for baby are vacuum and forceps delivery. When instrumental delivery is needed, baby can already have experienced a long labour and may have been caught in some very uncomfortable positions for a long period of time.

The use of epidurals has been shown to increase the rate of instrumental delivery as the urge to push can be somewhat reduced. After a long exhausting labour, it can be very difficult to get baby moving at this final stage before delivery.

Midwives and doctors will always monitor baby to ensure they are coping with labour and will only intervene when necessary. In recent years, forceps delivery has become less common. We still do see babies after a forceps delivery but more often, a vacuum delivery is the type of instrumental delivery we see. The more pushes with assistance that are required, the more likely it is that baby may be a little irritable after delivery. Sometimes only a "lift-out" is required, a little bit of help at the very end, as was the case for our older daughter. She was a vaginal birth after a previous C-section (VBAC) and was very unsettled that first night. She was born in St Thomas' Hospital in London and Rose's window overlooked Big Ben. She heard every hour ring out that night!

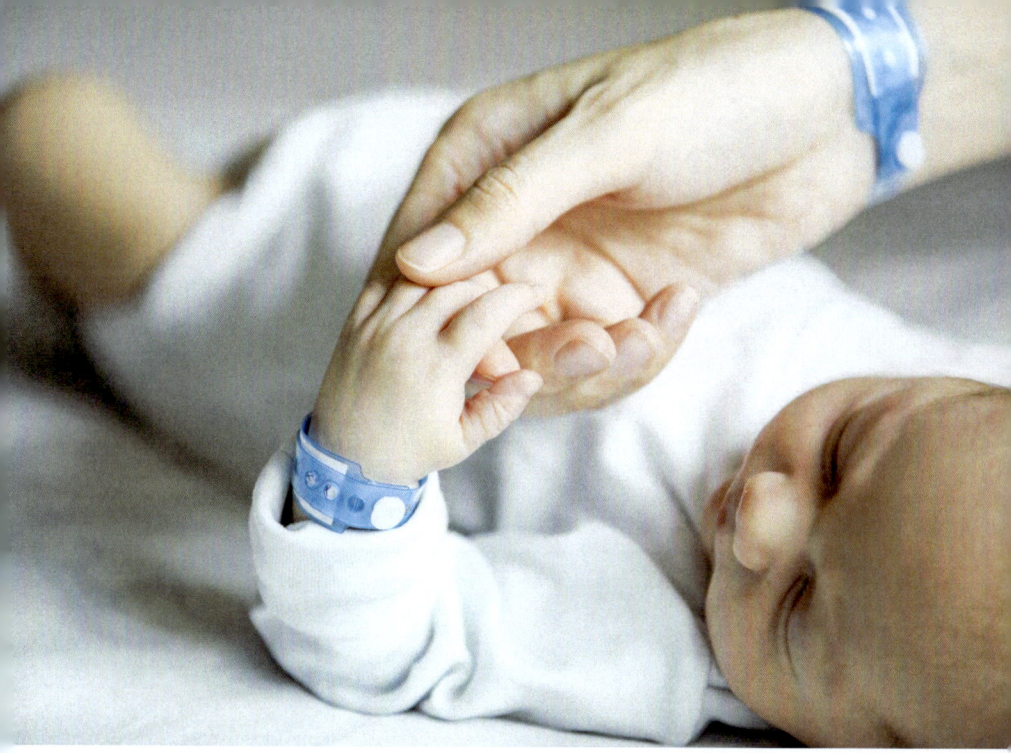

How a baby comes through the birth canal is also a contributory factor. Babies born in the occiput-posterior position (face up) often have a difficult time in labour as the largest diameter of the baby's head is leading the way. These labours can be longer too. We often see these babies for tight neck muscles on one side (torticollis), flattening of the head (plagiocephaly) or general irritability.

Sometimes at delivery a little hand or arm can present with the head. This can also cause issues with the neck and shoulder muscles.

Breech delivery is another high risk. However, most experts now recommend delivery by Caesarean-section (C-section) for all breech presentations. Having said all this, it's worth noting that babies can also have a very difficult delivery and sail through it without any problem at all. Every baby and delivery are different.

Another possible difficulty for babies is delivery by C-section, either planned or emergency. Our first baby was delivered by emergency C-section. He was very small for his dates and once labour started, he quickly became very distressed. Rose was a midwife working in the hospital he was born in and like any first-time parents, we had hoped for a normal delivery. Our little bundle was rushed to the Neo-Natal unit and for the first twelve hours all Rose had was a polaroid photograph of him. However, many C-sections are planned. These are less likely to have an undue effect on baby as everything is calm and labour has not started.

The main issue for a planned C-section baby is being delivered without being cleared of amniotic fluid. Babies born vaginally will have the benefit of having their chest cleared of amniotic fluid as they travel through the narrow birth canal and they then take that important first breath into clear lungs. With a C-section, this is not the case and as a result, baby can often be quite mucousy.

In cases where labour has begun and complications arise, baby may have travelled quite a way through the birth canal before a decision is made to perform an emergency C-section. They may have experienced a long labour before the decision to intervene for failure to progress, for example. This type of delivery can be difficult for baby as they will have both the labour and the C-section to deal with. They can be born in a state of shock and can be quite irritable in the first few days.

The length of labour is also important. Very long labours and very fast labours can affect baby. As baby comes through the birth canal, they turn in a corkscrew motion to adapt to the changing shape of the mother's pelvis. Doing this too slowly will result in baby being in very uncomfortable positions for long periods of time. Doing it too fast may result in baby born in a state of shock.

Depending on the circumstances, you can often have little control over how your baby enters the world. You can plan and prepare for labour and delivery, but sometimes, things don't go the way you intended. If a C-section is needed or an instrumental delivery is required, it is for the safety of you and your baby. If this happens it's important to remember that baby may need a little help afterwards.

Cranial osteopathy is a wonderfully gentle treatment that can help baby with the effects of any birth trauma or distress. Many midwives will recommend cranial treatment for babies who have had a tough time entering the world. In our experience, the sooner those stresses and strains are treated, the better for baby. Many babies we see are under six months old.

When parents bring their little one to see us, we take a detailed history of pregnancy and delivery. We ask about family history and about any medical interventions to date. Frank will ask about baby's feeding, sleeping, bowels and general wellbeing before deciding on a working diagnosis. He will then explain to the parents what is happening to baby so that they fully understand how they can help their little one. He may make some recommendations, about feeding perhaps, or a referral to another health practitioner. Baby is then treated. A follow-up appointment is required in most cases, to evaluate the treatment plan and to make any necessary changes to it.

It's never too soon to treat a baby after delivery. However, if baby is well, it's better to wait four weeks to allow feeding patterns to establish before considering cranial osteopathy treatment.

Martina's story

Like any new Mum, I was so excited about meeting my first baby. I felt I was prepared, having done classes about labour and delivery. I had a plan and my bags were packed. My labour started three days after my due date, and everything was ok at the start. I stayed home and walked around until the contractions become uncomfortable. We went to the hospital then but, after arriving, things slowed down.

After about eight hours the doctor suggested that I start on the drip to get things moving as I was only 3cms at that stage. I had really bad back pain and, as the contractions got stronger on the drip, it got very painful. I was so tired I decided to have an epidural. This helped for a little while. After a further five hours I had reached 9cms but baby was getting tired. I got to fully dilated and started pushing. This was so much harder than I imagined, particularly after such a long labour. Baby found the pushing very stressful and the doctor decided that a C-section was the best option. It was all very calm but quick in the end and my beautiful baby girl was delivered at last.

She was a little irritable for the first few days and one of the midwives suggested I bring her to see Frank as she had such a difficult labour and delivery. This was the best advice we got as the difference in her after just one treatment was amazing. She had a little frown after she was born, and my brother said she looked cranky! But Frank turned that frown upside down and the result was a very happy and contented baby and Mum.

The early weeks

The early weeks with a new baby are a magical time. Bringing baby home for the first time and getting to know your little one is what the early few days are all about. But it can also be a very busy and stressful time, particularly with the first baby.

When our first baby was born, we lived in London and had no family living in the UK. I guess because Rose was a midwife it was assumed that we would manage, and we did, but we were also new parents and Rose was recovering from a C-section. It was such a busy time as Frank started his osteopathy degree only a few days after our baby was born. That feeling of responsibility coupled with exhaustion and lack of sleep can feel overwhelming. This is a time of adjustment for everyone: for baby, for Mum and for Dad.

The adjustment for baby is centred around their change in environment from womb to world. This is a concept known as "The Fourth Trimester". Some babies make the transition very easily, others need a little more help. Understanding this and giving baby support while they make the transition to life outside the womb will make the process easier for both baby and parents. There are many things you can do to help baby during this time of change and development.

1. **Skin to skin contact** – Babies love skin to skin contact. The sooner you do this the better. Ask your midwife if you can have baby rest on your chest immediately after they are born. Doing this increases the levels of oxytocin, the love and bonding hormone. Skin to skin contact will regulate baby's heartbeat and stress hormones and is a wonderful way of calming baby during the early weeks.

2. **Movement** – Give anyone a little baby to hold and their first reaction is to sway from side to side. Babies love movement. There's an industry based on this, producing rockers, bouncers and swings.

3. **White noise** – When baby is in the womb they are continually subjected to quite loud white noise, so a quiet environment is very

uncomfortable for a newborn baby. Using white noise will calm baby by making them feel safe and secure and allows them to block out external stimuli when they are overwhelmed.

4. Slings – Slings are the ideal way to maintain the close contact your baby requires during the first few weeks. Babies have a feeling of security by being cocooned in a sling and have the added benefit of movement as you move around. There are many options available, so test a few before you decide which one suits you and your baby best. Maybe borrow some from friends or family before making your decision. Using a sling also means you are hands-free!

5. Swaddling – This is another way to give your baby a sense of security but there are safety precautions to be followed if you choose to do this. Only use a thin breathable fabric so that baby does not overheat. Learn the correct technique to swaddle your baby safely and do not swaddle if baby is unwell. Start swaddling early and discontinue once baby is three months old.

6. Bath – Up until birth, baby has been in a warm wet environment and a warm (not hot) bath will provide that floating feeling of the womb. This will calm and relax your baby and will become an important part of your night-time routine.

For Mum, everything changes in the blink of an eye when your baby is born. Having a baby is a life-changing event and the transition to motherhood can take time. During those first few weeks your new baby will need you constantly, 24 hours a day. You will be feeding, changing, soothing and rocking your baby while also recovering from the birth. You are at the mercy of your hormones and although you have been looking forward to this for a long time, it can feel overwhelming. But rest assured this is all very normal, you are not alone and you are doing a great job.

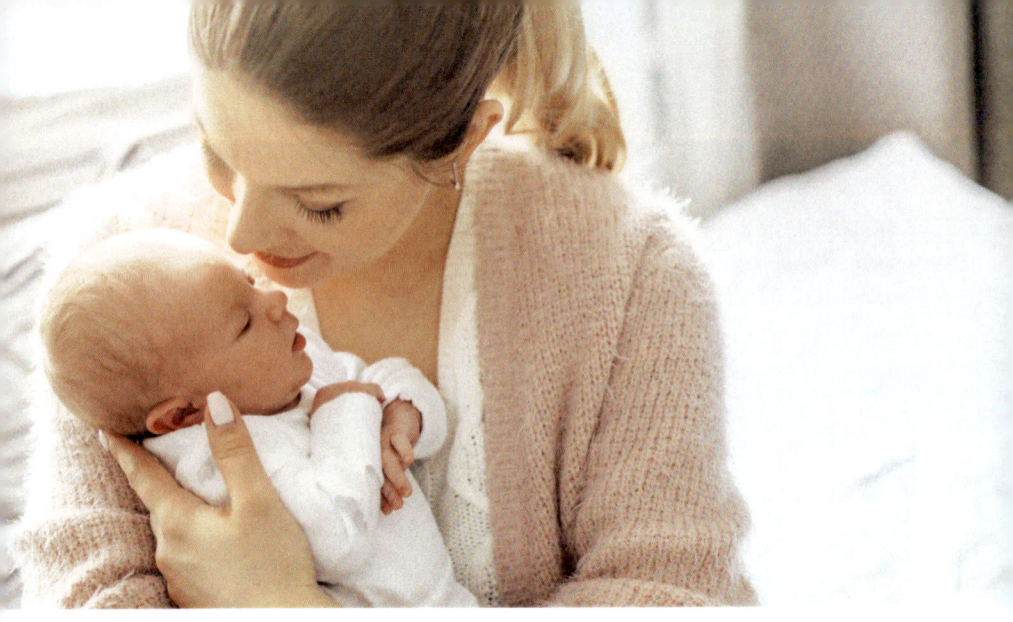

You may have more questions than answers at this time, but what you are doing is amazing, so remember that. Parenting can be difficult, and the struggles can sometimes overshadow the joy. There will be good days and not so good days but, as with everything, these too will pass. Allow yourself this "lying-in time" with your baby. Rest, bond and recuperate. Trust in your mothering instincts and remember that you are the expert on your baby, as you know baby best.

Dad too can need some time to adjust to this new role with all the responsibilities that it brings. Being the support for Mum during the early weeks is one of your most important jobs. Managing the daily tasks, other children and being the gatekeeper for enthusiastic visitors will allow Mum to cope with her job of looking after baby. Dad can also experience the magic of skin to skin contact with baby and by doing this, you can calm and bond with baby.

While baby spends most time with Mum, using the sling, swaddling and carrying baby are brilliant ways to give Mum a much-needed break. When Mum is breastfeeding, keep her hydrated and fed by getting her a drink and a healthy snack.

Remember you both are in this together. Support and encourage each other. And when things are difficult, remember that these moments will also pass, and you will all survive.

Infant reflux

The very word reflux can terrify parents of any small baby. In this chapter we will show you the many different types and levels of reflux and give you information to assist you recognise it, and all the treatment options. Armed with all this information, it will make your visit to your health practitioner a much more productive appointment. Giving them the right information allows them to get a better picture of what is going on and speeds up the diagnosis of reflux and consequently, the treatment.

What is reflux?

Reflux is a condition where the contents of the stomach pass into the oesophagus (food tube). This may then be swallowed back down (as in silent reflux), pass into the mouth (regurgitation) or be ejected from the mouth (vomiting).

Most new parents will not have heard of infant reflux and it may never enter their thoughts unless their baby presents with it. If you have had a baby with moderate to severe reflux, the word itself can raise your stress levels! Our first son had reflux, but thankfully not the painful type. He was a little early and quite small, so looking back now, it's not surprising.

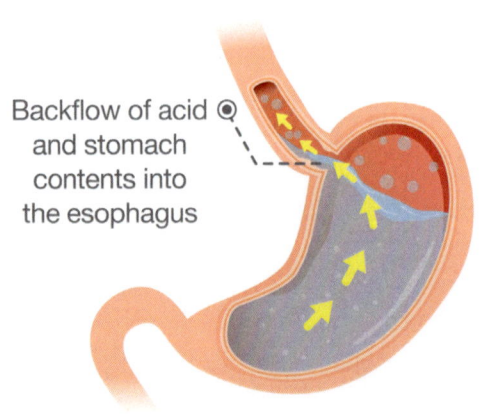

Backflow of acid and stomach contents into the esophagus

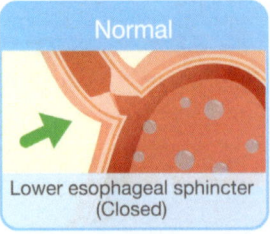

Normal

Lower esophageal sphincter (Closed)

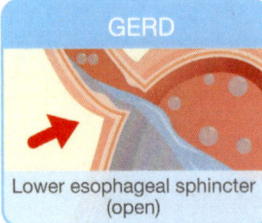

GERD

Lower esophageal sphincter (open)

Infant reflux is not uncommon and is not always necessarily a problem. Up to 70% of babies regurgitate some stomach contents into their mouth at least once daily. It is a normal occurrence and can be due to the frequency and size of baby's feeds putting the valve (sphincter) at the entrance to the stomach under pressure. This results in some stomach contents passing into the oesophagus or mouth. Remember a baby's stomach is only the size of their fist and their weight can triple in the first year of life. This growth requires constant feeding and can understandably put the stomach valve under a little pressure!

Remember that most babies regurgitate feed at least once a day. This is normal.

Reflux only becomes an issue when there are associated symptoms that cause distress. This is then called Gastro-Oesophageal Reflux Disease (GORD). This is the type of reflux that you hear all the stories about. In fact, books have been written just about this condition. While we feel we have given you enough information in this chapter, if your baby is on the severe end of the reflux scale, you may benefit from one of these books for a more detailed description of the condition.

Causes of GORD

There are two main causes of GORD: an under-developed lower oesophageal sphincter (valve), or a Cow's Milk Protein Allergy (CMPA).

The lower oesophageal sphincter

This sphincter or valve is located at the base of the oesophagus (food pipe) at the entrance to the stomach and its purpose is to keep the contents of the stomach where they belong. In some babies this valve can be weak or underdeveloped at birth, particularly if baby is a little premature. This can result in reflux.

As baby grows the valve will continue to develop and strengthen and, by the time baby is twelve months old, the valve will, in most cases, be much more effective. When baby is weaned to more solid foods, the contents of the stomach are thicker and more likely to stay where they belong rather than be regurgitated.

CMPA

It is estimated that up to 40% of babies with moderate/severe reflux disease have a CMPA. Many parents travel quite a way down the treatment road before a primary diagnosis of CMPA is even looked at. In our opinion, the sooner a CMPA is diagnosed the better the outcome for baby. The longer baby is exposed to an allergen, the more compromised their digestive and immune systems may become.

We see babies at the clinic who have struggled for months with a poorly managed reflux, secondary to an undiagnosed CMPA. Once weaning starts, the symptoms of reflux may become worse due to the overload of Cow's Milk Protein (CMP) in their system. These babies need the assistance of a paediatric dietician at this stage as they may also have developed other allergies. Nevertheless, with careful management these babies can be helped too.

If CMPA is confirmed by a paediatric dietician, dairy is removed from the diet and replaced with a suitable alternative. After time most children will be able to tolerate dairy again, although the re-introduction of dairy back into the diet must be managed carefully and under supervision of your dietician.

Very often, CMPA can also be seen in siblings. If one child has had reflux secondary to CMPA, it increases the possibility of subsequent children having reflux too. Once you have understood and managed reflux with a previous child, you will recognise the signs and symptoms earlier and in many cases the diagnosis is expedited, and the management plan can be put in place sooner.

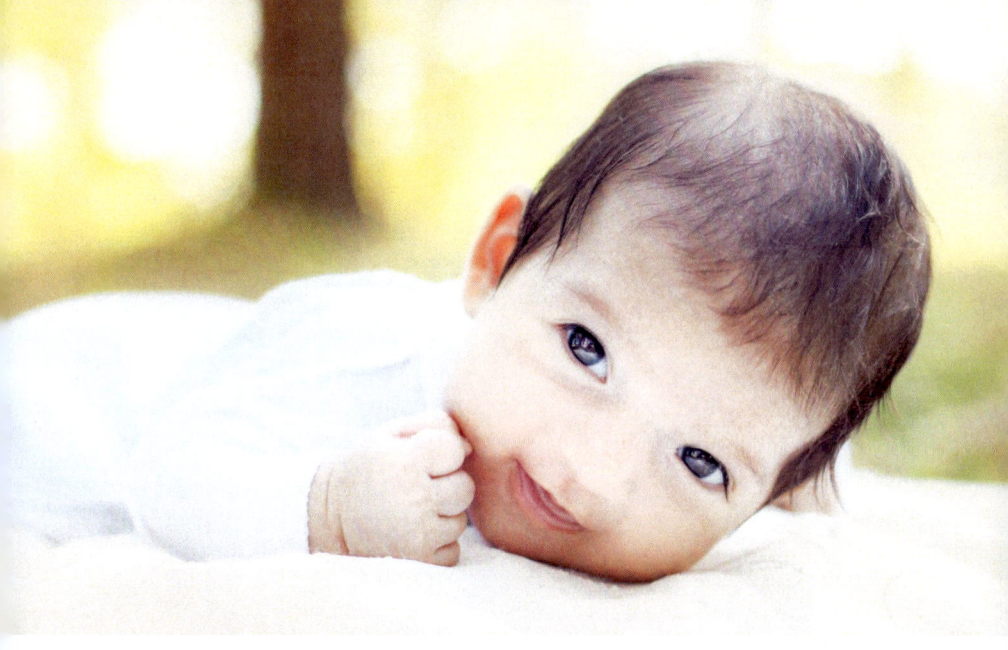

There are other conditions that may either cause reflux symptoms or mimic reflux symptoms and it's important to be aware of them as they should be considered if baby is not responding to treatment. These babies present with symptoms very similar to reflux. They may even have started treatment for reflux but get little or no relief from any of the different treatments and continue to be very unsettled.

The first condition is ***tongue-tie***. With this condition baby swallows too much air with the feed, both breast and bottle, as a result of reduced movement of the tongue preventing baby having a good latch on the breast or bottle teat. All the air in the tummy can push the feed out and mimic reflux. Until the tongue-tie is resolved, the symptoms will continue. You can read more about this condition in the chapter on tongue-tie.

Another condition is ***laryngomalacia***. This is a condition that is present at birth. During development, the supporting structures of the larynx do not develop fully. This results in floppy tissue above the vocal cords encroaching on the airway causing a stridor, or noisy breathing. The stridor associated with laryngomalacia is high pitched and more obvious when baby is breathing in, particularly during feeding and sleeping.

Feeding issues are common in babies with laryngomalacia as they have difficulty coordinating their breathing and feeding. This requires frequent breaks during feeding which can mean very long feeds, with some babies having trouble gaining weight. Some babies with more severe laryngomalacia also have reflux symptoms. In most cases, laryngomalacia is a harmless condition that will resolve naturally over time. If reflux is a concern, the baby is treated with medication. If sleep or feeding become very difficult, baby can have a small operation to remove the excess tissue from the larynx so as to allow easier breathing and swallowing.

The final condition is **eosinophilic oesophagitis**. This is an allergic condition of the oesophagus. It can happen at any age but in babies, it can present with signs and symptoms very similar to GORD. In this case the allergen could be a food such as CMP. During an allergic reaction, immune system cells gather and cause symptoms like redness, swelling and itchiness. A white blood cell called an eosinophil is one of these types of cells. Eosinophils are an important part of the immune system and there are always small quantities in the blood and intestine fighting parasites and performing other duties.

However, eosinophils cause problems when they appear in high quantities in areas other than the blood and intestine. In eosinophilic oesophagitis, eosinophils gather in the tissue of the oesophagus and cause redness, swelling and inflammation. This is a condition that was only discovered a few decades ago and cases seem to be on the rise in the last five years. If your baby is not responding to any of the treatments for GORD and if they are on the severe end of the reflux spectrum and are failing to thrive, it may be worth asking if eosinophilic oesophagitis is a possibility. Up to 10% of babies with severe reflux that is not responding to treatment are thought to have this condition.

Treatment involves identifying the food that baby has an allergy to and eliminating it from the diet. This is easier to do in babies under six months old as they have not yet been weaned and the food is likely to be milk.

TYPES OF REFLUX

There are four main types of infant reflux. Each has some similar signs and symptoms, and some have particular signs and symptoms that can help to identify it. In some cases, there may even be two types of reflux to manage.

Positional reflux

With this type of reflux baby spits up after a feed but is not very distressed by it. It can generally be resolved by keeping baby in an upright position during and after feeds. As stated earlier in this chapter, most babies spit up a little. Positional reflux is more than a little spitting up, sometimes referred to as a "happy spitter".Positional reflux

With this type of reflux baby spits up after a feed but is not very distressed by it. It can generally be resolved by keeping baby in an upright position during and after feeds. As stated earlier in this chapter, most babies spit up a little. Positional reflux is more than a little spitting up, sometimes referred to as a "happy spitter".

Silent reflux

With this type of reflux, the contents of the stomach are brought up but then swallowed back down. As a result, it can take a little longer to get a diagnosis, unless of course you know what other signs to look out for! These babies can be very distressed, and it is mostly by looking for the other signs and symptoms associated with silent reflux, that baby is diagnosed.

Acid reflux

Acid reflux is the most distressing type of reflux. The stomach contents that are regurgitated contain stomach acid that burns the ocsophagus, causing inflammation and pain. Think about what heartburn feels like yourself – that's what it's like for baby. These babies are often diagnosed early due to the high levels of distress involved.

Reflux secondary to CMPA

Very often reflux can be secondary to a CMPA. The severity of the reflux very often depends on the severity of the allergy. This type of reflux is also difficult to diagnose. Many parents will start off by treating the reflux symptoms. However, the reflux symptoms can be difficult to treat successfully while the allergy is not being addressed. The chapter on Cow's Milk Protein Allergy will give you a more detailed list of signs and symptoms for babies with a suspected CMPA.

> *A sling is a great way to keep baby upright after a feed for most reflux babies. Try out a few different slings before deciding which one suits you and your baby best. Perhaps borrow some from family or friends.*

It's important to seek medical assistance to determine which type of reflux is affecting your baby, as the treatment is different for each type. The list below is a guide for most of the possible signs and symptoms you may see. It's by no means an exhaustive list, but it will provide you with the information you need to give your medical practitioner so that they can make a quick and accurate diagnosis. If possible, bring a written list of signs and symptoms with you when seeing your doctor. This will ensure that you remember to tell your doctor everything. The symptom check list for reflux at the end of this chapter can be downloaded free from our website.

SYMPTOMS OF REFLUX

- Crying and irritability for longer than three hours a day. This can be at any time of the day or night.
- Regurgitation or vomiting of milk and/or clear fluid.
- Arching when feeding or after feeding.
- Wheezing on an ongoing basis.
- A noticeable breath change, where baby inhales and makes a gasping type of sound.
- Nasal congestion.
- Hiccoughs after most feeds. Many mums will also have been aware of baby having had hiccoughs in the womb.

Signs and symptoms specific to silent reflux

- Baby is continually swallowing and appears hungry when they're not.
- There is very little spitting up of feeds.
- Baby cries excessively.
- Baby seems to be in constant motion.
- Baby is very dependent on the upright position. Any change to a more horizontal position will not be tolerated well.
- Baby tends to comfort feed to reduce the symptoms.
- White milk can be observed coating the tongue.
- Silent reflux babies tend to like soothers.

Signs and symptoms specific to acid reflux

- Baby cries excessively. The cry is high pitched, and baby can often cry for up to six hours a day.

- Baby sweats excessively.
- Baby often refuses feeds. Baby may take the first part of the feed but once winded, will then refuse the remainder of the feed for up to 40 minutes after. They tend to graze on small amounts.
- There is very little relief from upright positioning.
- Baby is often in constant motion, using the motion to relieve the pain.
- Baby has chronic nasal congestion.
- Baby has chronic milk wheeze.
- Baby has a cough.
- Baby is likely to refuse a soother!

It's important to remember that baby will not have all these symptoms. This is a guide to help you recognise the general symptoms of reflux so that you can give your health practitioner as much information as possible.

MANAGEMENT OF REFLUX

Management of positional reflux

This is the mildest form of reflux and in most cases will resolve with a few simple measures.

Keep baby in an upright position if possible, during feeds and for at least 30 minutes afterwards. There are a number of slings and baby seats that you can get to help keep baby upright. One of our favourites is the Tiny Love Napper Rocker chair as the tilt can be adjusted to suit the needs of the baby. And of course, most babies love a sling. The benefit to Mum and Dad is that you have two free hands.

Gently wind baby frequently during the feed. Try a few different winding techniques. We suggest gentle rotation of baby's trunk while baby is sitting on your lap. Tilt baby back slightly and repeat the rotations. Rubbing the back rather than patting it is better for these babies.

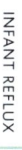

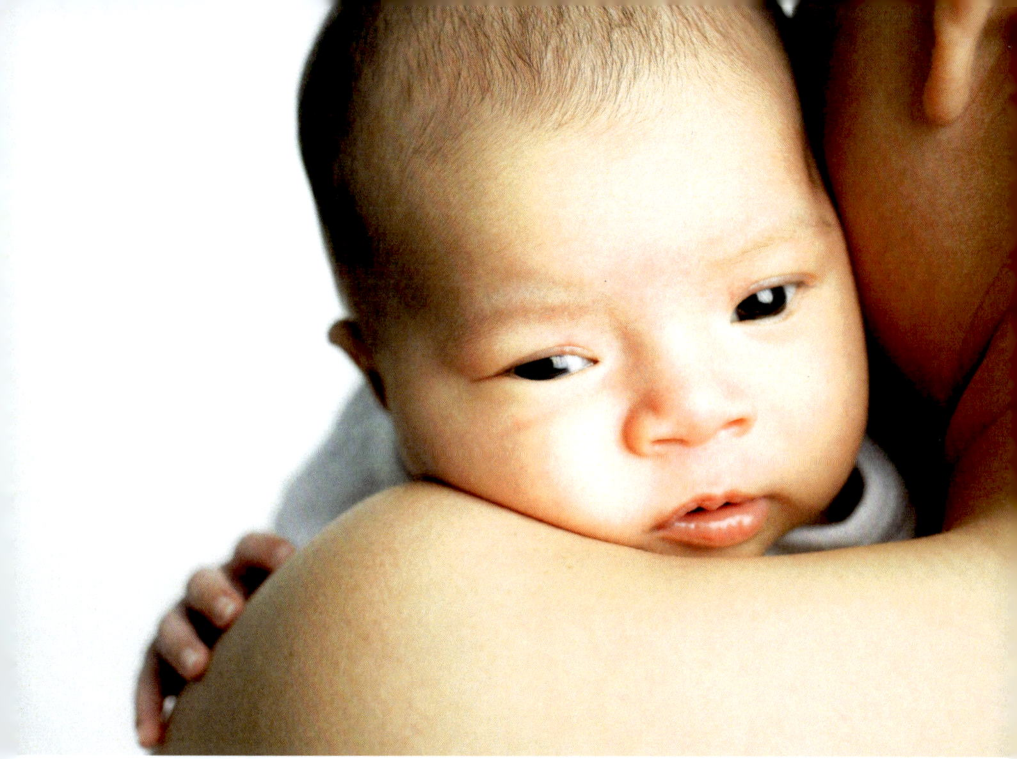

Do not overfeed baby. Monitor your baby's intake over 24 hours and avoid the temptation to give a little extra.

Gentle movement in a buggy may help so long as baby remains in the upright position.

Elevate the head of the cot so that baby is sleeping at a 30-degree tilt. You can buy cot elevators, or you can adapt something you have already to do the job. Just be sure that it's safe and secure.

If possible, never lie baby flatter than a 30-degree angle, even when changing a nappy. Change the nappy before a feed and only if needed after a feed when the tummy is full.

Avoid exposure to tobacco smoke as it causes irritability. This is a good idea for any baby but particularly for a reflux baby.

Avoid tight nappies or clothing, especially around the abdomen. Clothes with waistbands can be uncomfortable. A simple baby-grow will be best for baby but be aware of tight waistbands when you're dressing up little one for a trip out.

Management of silent reflux

You should use all the above techniques, plus, for a baby diagnosed with silent reflux, the following;

Gaviscon or Carobel are thickeners that can be used to thicken formula feeds. The reason for thickening the formula is to help keep it in the stomach. You should always follow the dosage guidelines on the packet, but you can adjust the amount of thickener downwards depending on your baby's needs.

When using a thickener, you should be aware that it may cause constipation. If this happens you can give baby some drinks of cool boiled water between feeds or/and you could reduce the amount of thickener in the feed. If this does not resolve the constipation you should discontinue the thickener and see your doctor.

A pre-thickened formula feed is another option. These feeds have a built-in thickener that starts to work once the formula is made up. You should follow the directions carefully as some formulas have very specific instructions for preparation. You will also find that you may need to move to a faster flowing teat so that baby can take the new formula easily. Using a regular size teat with a thickened formula will result in baby getting exhausted from the effort of sucking. They fall asleep and take less at each feed but wake after a short while looking for more food. Word to the wise, you should never add another thickener to an already pre-thickened formula.

> *Never use a thickening agent in a pre-thickened formula such as an anti-reflux formula.*

Babies with silent reflux very often fall into the category of acid reflux and may also require medication as discussed below.

Breastfed babies may also have silent reflux. It is certainly possible to treat a breastfed baby, but it is more of a challenge. When giving a thickener, you can use a little expressed milk in a teat and add the thickener to this. Give it before the breastfeed while baby is hungry. The advice of a lactation consultant may also be helpful and feeding baby in a more upright feeding position would be beneficial.

Infant Gaviscon: This is a thickening agent that contains sodium alginate and magnesium alginate. These ingredients form a gel in the stomach when they come into contact with the stomach acid.

Cow & Gate Carobel: This is a natural thickener which can be added directly to a formula feed.

Most thickeners are suitable for full-term babies and not recommended for premature or pre-term babies. Always follow the dosage guidelines, depending on the age of your baby. The dose can be adjusted downwards if baby gets a little constipated or as reflux resolves. Always consult your medical practitioner before starting use of a thickener.

Management of Acid reflux

You should look at all the above suggestions for a baby diagnosed with acid reflux in addition to speaking to your medical practitioner for advice regarding medications. Below are the most commonly used medications prescribed for babies with acid reflux.

Ranitidine (Zantac) – prescription only.

Zantac reduces the amount of acid in the stomach, which reduces the symptoms of acid reflux. Zantac comes in a liquid form for babies. Once opened, Zantac should be kept in the fridge and discarded after 4 weeks. The dosage of Zantac is based on baby's weight and should therefore be reviewed regularly with your doctor or pharmacist.

Very often we see babies who have done very well on Zantac initially only for symptoms to return after a few weeks. What has happened is that the reflux symptoms have improved, and baby had fed much better and put on weight. The dosage of Zantac initially prescribed may now not be enough, and symptoms return. Once the baby is weighed and the dosage of Zantac is reviewed by the doctor, baby improves again.

Zantac can taste quite sour so giving it with a little gripe water may help if baby does not like the taste. If baby tends to spit the Zantac back out at you, a quick but gentle blow of air into their face will make them swallow. Zantac can be given by syringe or in a bottle teat. It can be given over two or three doses a day.

Omeprazole (Losec Mups) – prescription only.

Losec is a Protein Pump Inhibitor (PPI) and blocks the production of acid in the stomach. Dosage is again based on baby's weight and should therefore be reviewed regularly with your paediatrician or doctor. If giving Losec twice a day, the evening dose should generally be given before 5.30pm as there is very little acid produced from 9pm till 2am (resting phase) and a PPI can only turn off a pump that is turned on.

During the resting phase there are very few acid pumps turned on and so, most of any dose given during this time will be of no use. From 2am to 7am there is an acid dump where the stomach produces extra acid. If your baby is most unsettled at night, then you could give the second dose of Losec at 12.30 to 1.30am.

Losec cannot be crushed and given with food. It must be dissolved in a little cold water and given in a syringe or off a spoon. For older babies the tablet can be dissolved in a little apple sauce. It is the beads you see after dissolving the tablet that contain the active ingredient. Losec should be given on an empty stomach and within half an hour of dissolving the tablet. A Losec tablet can be split in half using a splitter which your pharmacist can supply if the dosage requires this.

Management of reflux secondary to CMPA

Although it's important to follow the steps on the treatment ladder, it is also essential to be aware that when baby's reflux symptoms are not responding to treatment, the possibility of reflux being secondary to a CMPA must be considered.

A study done in Australia in 2008 stated that up to 40% of babies presenting with symptoms of GORD were diagnosed with a CMPA. If baby has any of the dermatological or respiratory symptoms associated with CMPA, it should be considered even sooner. The

> *Reflux is a condition that can vary from mild to very severe.*
>
> *If you have a baby with a severe reflux, do not be discouraged if someone gives you the simple solution that worked in two hours for their reflux baby and it doesn't work for your little one! Every reflux baby is different, and every day can also be different. Keep to the plan and have it reviewed often.*

reflux symptoms will be slow to improve while baby is still taking CMP. And in fact, if the CMPA is treated early on, the symptoms improve and you may not need to travel too far up the treatment ladder!

Read the chapter on CMPA in this book for more information and the presenting symptoms associated with an allergy to CMP. As with all the digestive disorders, you may find that you will be treating more than one condition at a time but, with information and support, that's very possible!

How can cranial osteopathy help a baby with reflux?

Cranial osteopathy, in a very gentle way, encourages the body's tissues to release any tension and increases tissue flexibility. Reflux in our opinion, challenges a number of key areas that support digestion. Firstly, the intestinal tract can become bloated and retain gas for longer periods. Secondly, the arching and extending associated with reflux can tension the breathing diaphragm as the baby is trying to ease their discomfort. Thirdly, as arching of the back persists, the neck musculature can also tension.

Treatment applied to these key areas allows a gentle releasing of tension and lengthening of these tissues. This creates a more comfortable feeding process for the baby and eases the tissues supporting digestion.

Reflux survival strategies

Infant reflux is a condition we see every day at the clinic. What our years of experience has shown us is that there are many different levels of reflux and there is no one solution that works for all babies. Some babies have a positional reflux, where keeping the baby propped up can alleviate the symptoms. Other babies have a mild acid reflux where a change of formula and perhaps an antacid will be the answer.

And then there are the babies with severe acid reflux! This is a completely different story. Caring for these babies can cause a significant amount of stress and distress. Treatment can include formula changes, medication and constant revisions, sometimes with very little success! Every day can be a challenge. With this in mind, we have listed a few tips for these parents specifically.

Don't expect to have all the answers at the beginning as it's a really steep learning curve. There will be plenty of well-meaning family and friends offering advice. Thank them but stick to the plan you have for your baby specifically.

There are no right or wrong answers for babies with reflux, as what works for one baby may not work for another. Take advice from your medical practitioner and ask as many questions as you need to, to understand your baby's condition. It really is trial and error until you find something that works for your baby.

When going to see your doctor with baby, write down all you want to tell or ask them. It's very easy to forget that very important question you wanted the answer for when you're sitting in front of the doctor and baby is crying. If possible, bring someone with you for support and assistance with baby. Our Symptom Checker is perfect for this.

Accept you are doing your best and focus on what's going right rather than what you feel is going wrong. Get everyone around you to buy into this too.

Believe in yourself and trust your instincts. Reflux is a complex medical condition; it's not in your head!

You can drive yourself crazy trying to figure out why one day is better or worse than another! The simple fact is that reflux can be cyclical, and some days may just be worse than others for reasons you may never know. Reflux can also get worse when baby is sick or teething. Don't blame yourself. Tomorrow may very well be a better day.

Look after yourself and accept any offers of help. Any Mum of a new baby may need help and having a reflux baby means you will very likely need help from family and friends. Please ask for help if you need it. Even asking for a meal for the freezer will be a help. Your family and friends will be looking for ways to make things easier for you. And if you feel things are getting on top of you, talk to someone – talking to someone can often relieve the strain and often helps you to see what you can do about the problem.

Many parents have reported that reflux can flare up when a baby is stressed or sick. Hot weather, teething, over-tiredness all can affect baby. However, knowing this can help as any changes make more sense.

Recognise that there will be times when you're more able to cope, and more positive, while other times you will feel quite low and overwhelmed. This is normal. Take each day as it comes and just maybe it helps to know that things will get better, no matter how hard it is right now. Remember though, that if you feel you're not coping, please ask for help and seek medical guidance. Your baby needs you to be well too.

Most reflux cases will settle in time, regardless of the severity. Some babies respond very quickly to treatment, while others take more time and more trial and error to get things right. There are many good books and apps available for the more severe type of reflux. There may also be a support group in your area or an online support group where you can get advice and encouragement from parents who are going through something similar.

The descriptions of the different types of reflux above will cover 95% of babies who present with reflux symptoms. There is however a very small percentage of babies who have ongoing, persistent and distressing symptoms and who will need close medical supervision and more detailed treatment.

Sarah's story

I brought my six-week-old baby to see Frank after a few very difficult weeks. She was crying and unsettled after most feeds and spitting up constantly. I had seen my doctor the week before and he prescribed her baby Gaviscon. It helped a little, but after a few days she ended up constipated.

Frank confirmed that Sarah had reflux. He told me that Gaviscon can sometimes make baby constipated and advised me to reduce the amount in each bottle. He gave me so many practical tips on managing the reflux by keeping Sarah upright.

I reduced the amount of Gaviscon in Sarah's feeds after the visit to Frank and kept her propped up for a good hour after her feeds. She was still spitting up a little, but she didn't seem to mind it. Her constipation resolved and she started smiling again. We returned two weeks later with a much happier baby. Sarah was feeding, winding and pooing better and was at last enjoying her feeds. It certainly helped to keep her upright too. We still get moments when she is upset, but nothing like how she was before.

Thomas's story

Thomas attended the clinic at five weeks old. He was born at 40 weeks and 3 days after a 24-hour labour. Mum stated that after about eight days she started to notice that Thomas was crying more often during and after feeds, he was drinking his bottles very quickly, winding him had become more difficult and he was re-swallowing what appeared to be clear liquid with milky bits in it about an hour after his feeds. He was vomiting up milk once a day only. He was also congested and was coughing more often to clear his throat.

Mum had taken Thomas to the Public Health Nurse and she recommended a change to a comfort formula and to monitor his symptoms. Mum also attended her doctor who diagnosed reflux and Thomas was prescribed Zantac. These changes had made some difference to Thomas, but he was still very irritable.

On case history examination using a symptom checklist, I diagnosed Thomas with silent reflux. I treated his upper digestive system to give him relief. Silent reflux requires various supports to manage the condition effectively. It is important to ensure that the formula is the correct density to reduce regurgitation. Also, the medication should be reviewed every couple of weeks with the doctor to ensure it is working, based on the baby's increased body weight. Elevation and sleeping position are very important in retaining the contents in the stomach as the baby can have heartburn episodes due to regurgitation.

I advised Mum about these key areas. The management is effective if you apply these changes and use our Symptom Management Chart (available to download free from our website) to closely monitor your baby for progress. Review everything regularly and be objective. With these changes Thomas improved significantly. He still had episodes of reflux, but the frequency reduced and Mum managed them much better.

Michael's story

Michael was an eight-week-old baby when his Mum brought him to the clinic. She stated that Michael's level of crying significantly increased from two weeks old. He was in pain when burping, going quite rigid and red-faced. He was looking to feed every two hours and was unable to lie down flat in his crib. Most feeds had become difficult to finish and he was taking 2–3ozs at a time and then refusing to continue to feed.

Mum had been to her doctor and Public Health Nurse several times. On their recommendation, Michael had changed formula from standard to comfort and was now on an anti-reflux formula. Michael was also on a medication for reflux. At the beginning, each change had made a difference to Michael's distress but, after several days his symptoms returned.

On case history taking, Mum stated that Michael was experiencing pain during and after feeding, bloating, bowel variability, constant feeding, nasal congestion and regurgitation. As a result of this Michael was very wakeful all day and only sleeping in an upright position at night. On further questioning I asked Mum about Michael's skin condition. She said that he had several rashes that would come and go. His skin was dry on the face, limbs and chest. He was developing cradle cap. There was a family history of food intolerance to diary as two of Michael's first cousins were on special formulas as babies.

My conclusions, having spoken to Mum and examined Michael, and having looked at other factors, was that Michael could have a CMPA. His reflux wasn't responding to treatment because the underlying issue was intolerance. I treated Michael at the clinic to ease his digestive system.

I referred Michael back to his doctor. Michael was prescribed a dairy-free formula and within a week his symptoms started to improve significantly, but he still had periods where his reflux was active. I explained to Mum that this can be the case and provided her with practical tips on how to manage these episodes.

I re-evaluated Michael at the next visit based on our Symptom Management Chart I had given Mum to fill out to monitor Michael's progress. He was much improved and was discharged with a follow-up in a month.

REFLUX SYMPTOM CHECKER

SYMPTOM

Crying and irritability for more than three hours

Regurgitation of milk

Regurgitation of clear fluid

Arching when feeding or after feeding

Wheezing on an ongoing basis

Nasal congestion

Hiccoughs

Baby continually swallowing

Baby comfort feeds

Baby is in constant motion

White milk can be seen on the tongue

Baby sweats excessively

Baby refuses feeds

Baby has a cough

Baby is not gaining weight

Tick if your baby has this symptom

Use this chart to document your child's symptoms. When you go to see your health professional, bring your Symptom Checker with you as this will be helpful in assisting them to make a diagnosis. It also ensures that you will remember to tell your health professional everything!

At the back of this book you will find a Symptom Management Chart. By observing and grading five key areas you will get a broad picture of how baby is doing over a full week. This allows you to record the various symptoms to allow your medical practitioner to look at them objectively. Both these charts are also available to download free from our website.

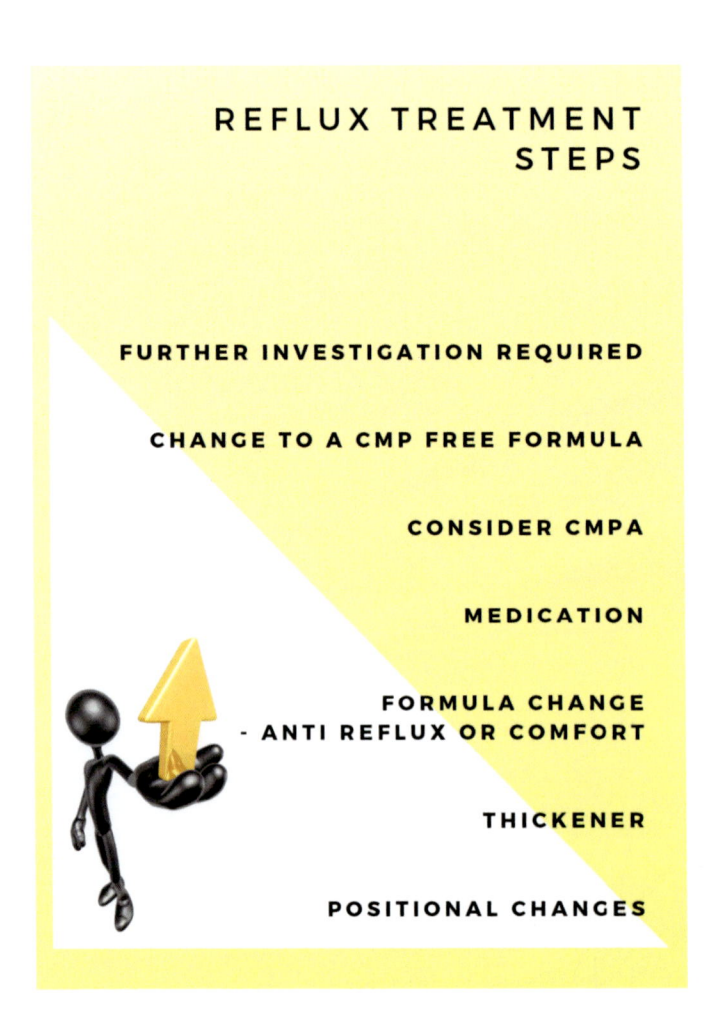

REFLUX TREATMENT STEPS

FURTHER INVESTIGATION REQUIRED

CHANGE TO A CMP FREE FORMULA

CONSIDER CMPA

MEDICATION

FORMULA CHANGE - ANTI REFLUX OR COMFORT

THICKENER

POSITIONAL CHANGES

Lactose overload

Although lactose overload and colic are very similar conditions, we believe they both deserve their own chapter. Lactose overload is mostly a breastfeeding issue, but we have also seen it in formula fed babies. Colic, on the other hand, is an over-used term to describe a collection of problems all involving a crying, unsettled baby. There are varying theories about colic, and we have one too. If you feel your baby may have colic, please read this chapter on lactose overload as it may better explain what is happening and why your little one is distressed.

Some medical practitioners refer to lactose overload as colic. While they are comparable, we think otherwise.

Lactose is the sugar found in breast milk and most formula feeds. It's a disaccharide molecule made up of one unit of glucose and one unit of galactose, which are joined together by a chemical bond. However, in this form, lactose cannot be digested, so it must be broken down into its two digestible parts – glucose and galactose. This happens in the small intestine, where an enzyme called lactase is produced. Lactase splits the bond joining glucose and galactose.

Lactose sugar is the main source of energy for most babies and all babies produce the enzyme lactase, with extremely rare congenital exceptions. Lactase is produced in the small intestine at a slow and steady rate, regardless of the level of lactose sugar present. When the gut gets overloaded with lactose sugar, baby will begin to show symptoms of lactose overload.

Lactose overload, or secondary lactose intolerance, is a condition we see in babies when either: too much lactose (sugar found in milk) is ingested, there is an overly fast gastric clearance, or there is a reduced amount of the enzyme lactase produced in the small intestine.

It's important to understand why each of these happen so let's look at each of them in detail.

Too much lactose sugar ingested

In bottle-fed babies who take high volumes of formula feeds we can often see some of the signs and symptoms of lactose overload.

The volume of lactose sugar arriving in the gut is too much for the baby's digestive system to manage. Some of the lactose sugar is broken down by the available lactase enzyme but some is not.

Many babies will get a few hours towards the end of the day where they are unsettled. You'll find yourself walking around with baby in your arms trying to soothe them. It's very likely that lactose overload may account for this upset in some babies. Of course, over-stimulation of the nervous system may also be a factor. Unfortunately, this upset happens at what is a busy time in most homes when dinner and bath-time for other children is happening too.

In breastfed babies the main issue causing too much lactose sugar in the diet is oversupply of breast milk. In this instance, baby fills up very quickly at the beginning of the feed and often does not get to the high-fat hindmilk, a crucial part of the breast feed.

Fast gastric clearance

This is exclusively a breastfeeding issue. The hindmilk is the high-fat breast milk that baby gets towards the end of a breastfeed. The fat in the hindmilk slows down the transit of feed thru the baby's gut, allowing time for the lactase enzyme to break down the lactose sugar. Babies who do not get enough of this high-fat hindmilk have a faster gastric clearance. This means that a high proportion of lactose is not broken down into its two digestible parts. This sets off a different series of events in the gut.

Reduced production of the enzyme lactase

The Brush Border in the small intestine contains the cells that produce the enzyme lactase. This area may become damaged due to an allergic reaction to cow's milk protein (CMP). The result is a temporary reduction in the amount of lactase enzyme produced. Consequently, there can be high levels of undigested lactose sugar in the gut.

Signs and symptoms

In a bottle-fed baby
- Gassy baby
- Irritable and crying, pulling his legs up
- Watery nappies
- Sore bum

In a breastfed baby
- Gassy baby
- Irritable and crying, pulling his legs up
- Frequent, green, watery nappies
- Mucousy stools
- Sore bum

To fully appreciate how this condition can affect your baby it's important to understand why the signs and symptoms occur.

Gassy baby. Excessive undigested lactose sugar in baby's gut is fermented by the gut flora to produce gases and acid. This causes lower bowel pain with baby drawing up his legs and crying. This is different to a windy baby where the gas is in the stomach. When a baby has lower gut gas you can hear the baby groaning with it. Very often we hear these babies groaning in the clinic before they go into Frank's treatment room. We know they have lower gas just by the sounds they make. Baby will also pass wind but can be quite uncomfortable with lower gut gas.

Frequent, explosive, watery yellow/green stools. The products of lactose fermentation (gases and acid) and the remaining undigested lactose in the baby's gut prevents water in the gut from being absorbed and draws extra water into the intestines. In breast-fed babies a feed that has a low-fat content will also speed up the transit of food thru the baby's gut. The result can be frequent, watery stools that are yellow/green in colour.

Mucousy stools. In breast-fed babies, depending on how quickly the gastric clearance occurs, there may be mucus in the baby's stools also.

Irritability and crying. Baby can be very irritable due to the discomfort felt as a result of the over-production of intestinal gases. Another factor for breast-fed babies, which only aggravates the problem, is that due to the fast gastric clearance, baby can often show signs very quickly that they are hungry again. The sucking action may give a little relief by dispersing some of the gastric gases. However, another feed arriving into an already compromised gut may only make things worse!

Sore bum. Depending on the severity of the lactose overload, some babies experience a nappy rash due to the presence of acid in the stools (one of the products of lactose fermentation).

Management and treatment of lactose overload

Management of lactose overload will be decided by the primary cause and may require a little trial and error, as all babies are individual. It's always a good idea to speak to a health professional about your baby.

Your lactation consultant, doctor or public health nurse will be able to advise you on what's causing the condition and direct you towards the correct treatment option. We now describe what we advise parents to do, based on the primary cause of lactose overload.

If baby is taking too much milk

Every baby is different, and some babies will require more or less feed than others. In bottle-fed babies it's easy to see how much baby is taking. The chart below gives you an idea of how much formula baby should be taking. The general rule is 2.5oz of formula for every pound (1lb) of your baby's body weight per day. For example, a 13lb baby will consume around 32oz of formula milk in any 24 hours.

The successful management of lactose overload must firstly identify the primary cause of the condition, as this will determine the treatment.

The chart below applies if baby is more than one week old, is a healthy full-term baby and is not yet eating solids. Remember there are always babies who will take a little more or a little less than the average below, so it's only a guide.

1–4 WEEKS
In the first few weeks of life a baby's tummy is very small and unable to hold large amounts of milk at a time, so they will need to feed on small amounts often. Most newborn babies will consume somewhere between 30–60mls (1–2oz) each feed, eating 8–10 times in a 24-hour period.

1 MONTH
By the time your baby is one month old, he/she will probably want between 90mls (3oz) and 120mls (4oz) at each feed. They'll consume anywhere from 400mls (13.5oz) to 800mls (27oz) in one day. Once your baby finishes a bottle without any encouragement and starts searching for seconds you will know his appetite is growing.

2 MONTHS
At two months your baby will want between 120–180mls (4–6oz) at each feed and will feed about 6–8 times a day.

3–6 MONTHS
Babies in this age group will typically want 4–5 feeds a day with around 180–200mls (6–7oz) at each feed. This might swap to 3–4 feeds with about 200–220mls (7–8oz) as they reach closer to their six month birthday.

If you feel your baby is taking more than the amounts above, you should discuss possibly changing to a hungrier baby formula with your public health nurse. You can also add lactase drops to your baby's feed. These drops act in the same way as the enzyme lactase. They start to work immediately and can take the pressure off a very busy gut.In breastfed babies it's a little different. Many parents worry that their baby is not getting enough milk. In fact, this is one of the main reasons why mothers stop breastfeeding. However, the truth is that most breastfeeding mothers have a perfectly adequate milk supply.

A good idea is to use your baby's output as an assessment tool to determine if your baby is getting enough breast milk. After all, what goes in must come out. The chart below shows you what's normal for breast-fed babies from day one to day six and beyond. Again, remember that every baby is different, and this is just a guide.

DAY	NUMBER OF WET NAPPIES	NUMBER OF DIRTY NAPPIES	STOOL COLOUR
1	1	1	Black tarry
2	2	2	Brown/black tarry
3	3	3	Greenish
4	4	3–4	Greenish/yellow
5	5–6	3–4	Yellow
6+	5+	3–4	Yellow

By observing your baby's output, you will be able to recognise when your baby's intake is either too low or too high and get the help of a lactation consultant to get you back on track.

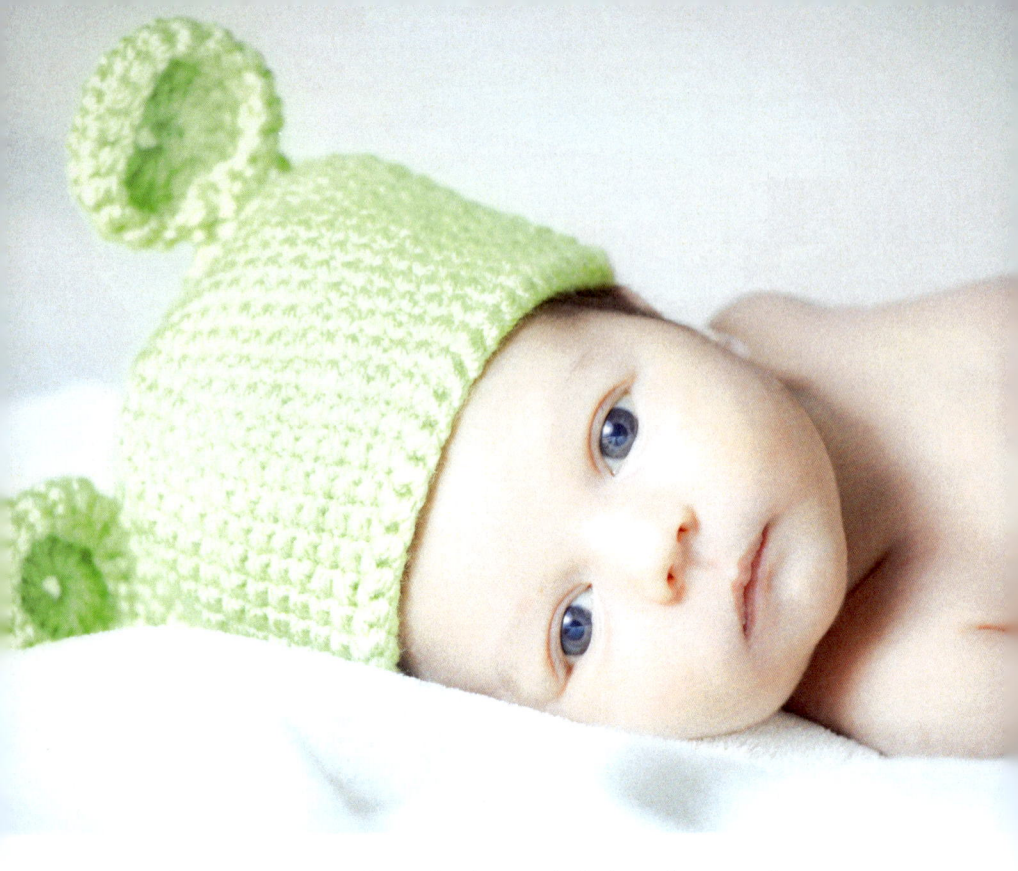

Sometimes a mother who is worried about her supply may over-compensate by offering more feeds than baby needs and by doing so may over-stimulate her supply. The advice and help of a lactation consultant can very often be the thing that keeps a mother breastfeeding when she would otherwise have given up. If you have any concerns about your baby's output, ask for help early.

Lactase drops

These are drops that can be purchased at your pharmacy. They are an artificial form of the enzyme lactase and work in the same way by breaking milk sugar (lactose) into its two digestible parts. They can be added to some formula feeds where they start working straight away.

Lactase drops can also be used for breastfed babies. They will supplement the baby's own supply of the enzyme lactase and help with the important work of breaking down lactose into glucose and galactose. To give these drops, a breastfeeding mum should start the feed for 2–3 minutes and then remove baby from the breast. Apply the drops directly onto the nipple and re-attach baby. It's that simple!

Fast gastric clearance

This is something that only happens in breast-fed babies. The hindmilk is the later part of a breastfeed. Allowing a baby to drain one breast before offering the second breast will ensure that baby receives both foremilk and hindmilk during the feed. The main reason fast gastric clearance occurs is a lack of high fat hindmilk in the breast feed. Fat will slow down the passage of food through the gut allowing time for lactase enzyme to break down the lactose sugar into its two digestible parts. Without the fat of the hindmilk, the passage of food through the gut will be speeded up.

There are many reasons a breast feed can be low in the high fat hindmilk:

- Shortened breastfeeds due to sore nipples/breast.

- Poor positioning or attachment resulting in a poor sucking action by baby. The feed can take a long time and baby can get too tired to finish.

- Babies who are fed according to the clock rather than by being baby-led are more likely to get a lower amount of hindmilk. For example; ten minutes each side four hourly.

- Tongue-tie. This can also affect the baby's latch and result in long ineffectual feeds. For more information see the chapter on tongue-tie.

- Infant oral thrush can also reduce the effectiveness of the suck and the feed.

Most breastfeeding issues can be dealt with very effectively by getting the advice of a lactation consultant sooner rather than later. Breastfeeding can be overwhelming when things are not going to plan, and a lactation consultant will be able to get you back on track. Many maternity units also offer breastfeeding support groups. Again, ask for help as it may make the difference between continuing breastfeeding and giving up.

> *If a breastfeeding mum's diet is low in fat and high in sugar her breastmilk can be higher in lactose and lower in fat! As you can now see that will have implications in the digestive tract of your baby. Try not to skip meals or snack on high sugar foods. Instead eat a well-balanced diet and always try to have a good breakfast. If family or friends ask what they can do to help, ask for a meal for the freezer.*

Damage to the lactase producing cells

This can occur in both bottle and breastfed babies and is a result of an allergy to CMP in the baby's diet. In our opinion, there are varying degrees of sensitivity to CMP. In babies who have sensitivity to CMP, the cells that produce the enzyme lactase are damaged by an allergic response to the protein. This results in less enzyme being produced by the cells, causing a lactose overload in the gut.

In breast-fed babies our recommendation is to remove CMP from the mother's diet for twenty days. If baby has a CMP sensitivity, he will show a significant improvement over the twenty days. In this case CMP should be removed from the mother's diet for a period of six weeks to allow the lactase producing cells to recover. It may be beneficial to consult a dietician to ensure you are maintaining a healthy diet.

After a period of time, you can test baby's reaction to CMP again by Mum taking a small amount of CMP in her diet and monitoring baby's response to it over the next 2–3 days. If any symptoms return, then it's safe to assume that baby is not ready for CMP yet and it should be removed from the mother's diet again. Remember also that it is always best to see a paediatric dietician for advice and support around weaning if you think your little one may have a CMPA.

In bottle-fed babies, it's a little more complex! There's a sliding scale of sensitivity to CMP in bottle-fed babies and the best formula is the one that matches your baby's level of sensitivity. It's important to remember that although baby is experiencing the symptoms of lactose overload, the main cause is a CMP sensitivity. This is the condition that must be treated first.

By changing the type of protein or removing CMP from your baby's diet you are allowing the cells that produce the enzyme lactase time to recover. This can take up to six weeks. During this time, you must also treat the lactose overload. The treatment will be determined by how sensitive your baby is to CMP and by which formula is best suited to your baby's needs.

For example; *Aptamil Pepti* is a formula that contains lactose and in which the CMP has been extensively broken down. This would suit a baby with a mild sensitivity. However, as it contains lactose, you would also have to use lactase drops for a period of six weeks while the gut heals.

Nutramigen is a similar formula in that it also has extensively broken-down proteins, but it is lactose free. If you were using this formula, you would not need lactase drops. If, however, your baby is more sensitive to CMP, this formula may not suit, and baby may require a CMP-free formula.

Another suggestion to assist the compromised gut is probiotics. Always use a dairy free probiotic which will re-establish a robust and balanced gut flora. You can read more about the benefits of probiotics in the next chapter on colic and gut health.

When your baby has more than one digestive condition it may take slightly more time to find a solution. You should always consult a medical professional to ensure your baby is receiving the correct treatment.

Ben's story

Ben was my second baby and having breastfed my first, I felt very confident this time round. The first few weeks went as expected but, by week three, Ben was having long periods of time when he was very unsettled. By dinner time it was usually chaos in our house with a crying baby and everyone hungry. I was constantly changing his nappies too and they were so runny and offensive.

I brought him to see Frank as I had brought my first child and the treatment had really helped him settle. Frank said that Ben was becoming overloaded with milk sugar towards the end of the day and explained how this was causing all his issues. He suggested giving him lactase drops during the day to take the pressure off his gut. He treated him and told me to come back if I needed to.

I started the drops that day and I started to see an improvement straight away. After about three days Ben was so much better. On Frank's recommendation, I attended the hospital breastfeeding support clinic to be sure my feeding techniques were good. Got top marks there but was very happy I went as I met a few other mums who were also breastfeeding and we met up for coffee the following week.

LACTOSE OVERLOAD SYMPTOM CHECKER

SIGNS & SYMPTOMS	BREAST-FEEDING	BOTTLE-FEEDING
Gas and bloating		
Frequent explosive stools		
Green stools		
Watery stools		
Mucousy stools		
Irritability and crying		
Sore bum/nappy rash		

Use this chart to document your child's symptoms. When you go to see your health professional, bring your Symptom Checker with you as this will be helpful in assisting them to make a diagnosis. It also ensures that you will remember to tell your health professional everything! You can get a free download of this chart on our website.

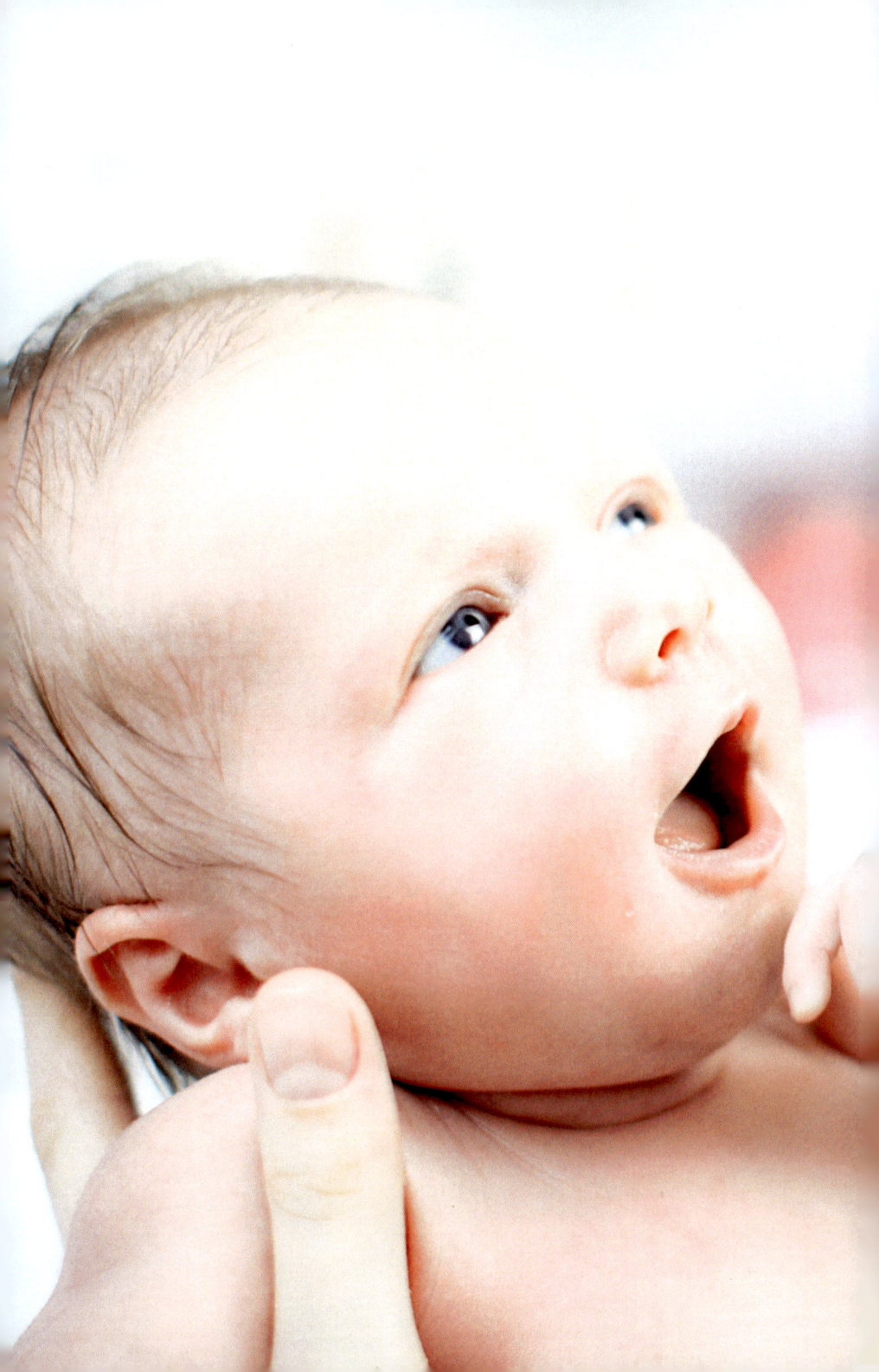

Colic and Gut Health

According to most health professionals, about 20% of babies develop colic. There is a generally accepted rule of three – if your baby cries inconsolably for more than three hours a day, more than three days per week and is aged between three weeks and three months, he may be diagnosed with colic.

A classic case of colic is where the baby pulls his knees up, clenches his fists, closes his eyes tightly or opens them wide. They may even hold their breath for a short time. Bowel activity increases, and your baby may pass "wind".

However, colic is a term that is used widely by people who do not have another reason for baby's distress. In our experience, there is more likely to be a cause for little one's distress rather than it being a case of true colic. Therefore, it's always wise to look at other digestive issues that can affect baby before deciding it is colic.

Over the years we have noticed that when a baby presents with colic-type symptoms, and we have ruled out other digestive issues, the most likely cause is a gut immaturity or imbalance.

Many of the bacteria in a newborn baby's gut come from Mum. The type of delivery is important in determining how populated the baby's gut will be with good bacteria. A vaginal birth exposes the baby to the mother's vaginal microflora and allows the baby's gut to be well populated by good bacteria. A baby delivered by C-section is delivered into a sterile environment. This can therefore affect the level of good bacteria in the gut. This small difference, resulting from different types of delivery, has been shown to have an influence on the development of a healthy immune system.

In some countries they have started to intervene in this process for mums having a planned C-section. Prior to the surgery a piece of gauze is inserted into the Mum's vagina and after the baby is delivered, the gauze is removed and the baby is wiped down with it. This process simulates the exposure that would happen in a vaginal delivery and no doubt goes some way towards increasing the level of good bacteria in the baby's gut.

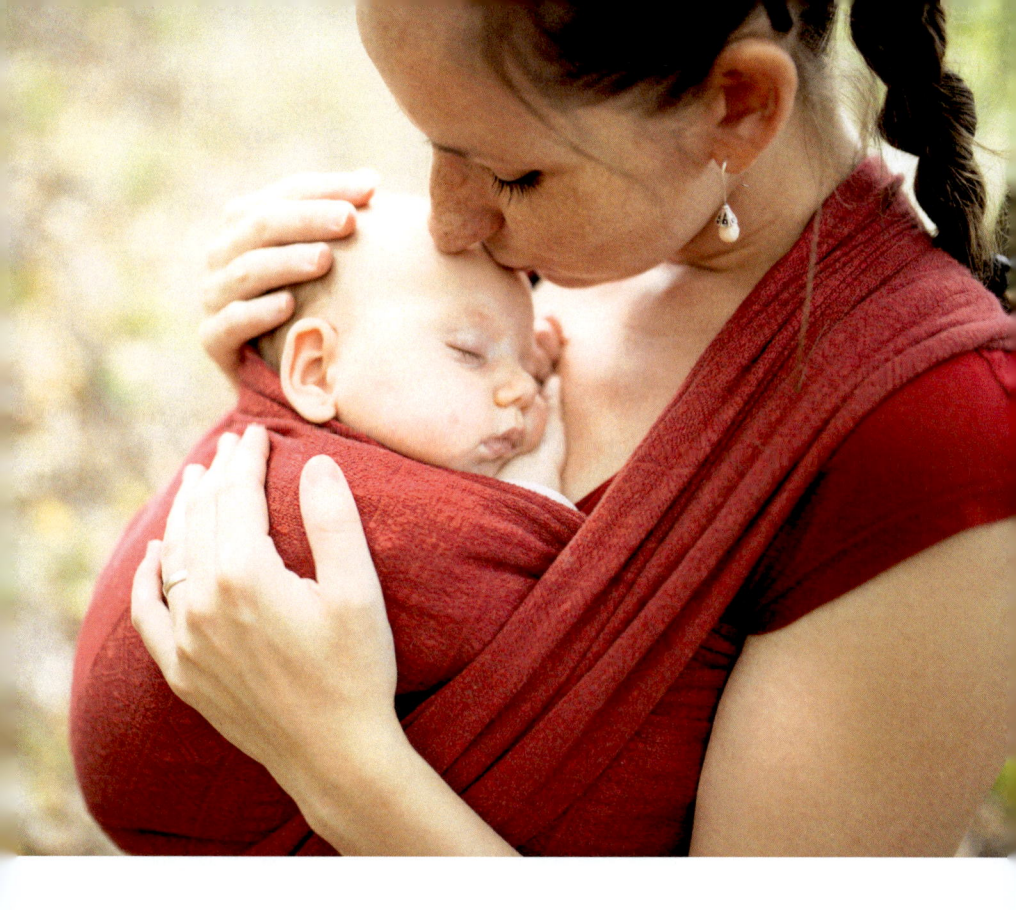

We must also factor in gut maturity. It's worth remembering that anything from 38 weeks to 42 weeks of pregnancy is considered to be full-term. That's a four week difference between two full-term babies and a four week difference in gut maturity.

The next thing that influences the gut health is how a baby is fed. In the first year of life, 30% of breastfed babies' gut bacteria comes from breast milk and a further 10% from the Mum's breast. This is another reason why support for breast feeding mothers is so valuable, particularly following a C-section. Many of the formula companies have now included prebiotics to their infant formulas to try to address this imbalance. If a baby has antibiotics at any stage this too will negatively influence the gut health.

How to solve colic

We see babies who have issues with their gut health or their gut development at our clinic every week. They present with typical colic-type symptoms, grunting and straining with lower gas and can be generally unsettled. The main aim of our treatment is to give their gut a little help.

Firstly, we suggest an infant probiotic. This should be used daily for six weeks. The probiotic we generally recommend is Proven. It has both breastfed and bottle-fed products and its breastfed version is dairy free. However, any good pharmacy will have an infant probiotic. Speak to the pharmacist for advice regarding which one is best for your baby.

The second thing we suggest is lactase drops. These are an artificial form of the enzyme that is produced in the small intestine to break down milk sugar. This enzyme is produced at a slow and steady rate in the gut. Many babies can struggle towards the end of the day when the demand for this enzyme is high and this results in some milk sugar left undigested in the gut. Bacteria work on this free sugar and one of the byproducts is gas. This gas can cause pain and distress for your little one as they wriggle and strain to release it. Did you know that 95% of digestion occurs in the small intestine? That is why a healthy gut is so important in babies.

The combination of probiotics and lactase drops has been very successful in babies with colic over the years. This magic duo has helped many babies go from a distressed crying baby to a happy smiling one.

Some bottle-fed babies can take in too much air when feeding and this can cause distress. Every baby is different and what suits one baby will not necessarily suit another. However, if you feel your little one is taking in air with the feed or does not have a good latch on the teat of the bottle, then a change of bottle and teat type would be recommended. We recommend MAM bottles for these babies. The surface area of the teat is much larger, and this increases the contact baby has with the teat. The better the contact, the lower the risk of taking in air.

There are specific formulas on the market for babies with colic. These comfort formulas contain partially broken-down milk proteins and a reduced amount of lactose milk sugar. As you can now see, these formulas would suit best if baby's symptoms are more as a result of a lactose overload. As with many digestive conditions, there can be an overlap, so you should always speak to your health practitioner before you change formula.

Premature babies seem to be more likely to have immature gastrointestinal systems. We see these babies in our clinic after they are discharged from hospital and on regular formulas. In our experience, a change to an organic formula, in addition to some of the other treatment options, brings about a significant change.

Some babies with colic like to be held in the "Tiger in the Tree" position. Support your baby by lying him across your arm facing downwards with his head near your elbow. Support his weight with your arm while holding a leg.

Another theory is that colic may be as a result of nervous system over-stimulation. We hear from parents so often about how colic seems to start in the early evening. They tell us that the more they try to soothe their baby, the more distressed baby can become. We have often advised these parents about cutting down on external stimuli and have suggested a little siesta for baby just before the early evening upset. The feedback has been very positive with parents reporting that baby was better able to cope with the evening period by giving baby a little time to rest their brain and nervous system. Again, all babies are different and they respond to different things, but this may be worth a try. Read about other ways to calm your baby in the chapter on "The Early Weeks".

Tips for colic

- Breastfeeding mothers should avoid spicy or heavy foods. Dairy products, broccoli, cabbage, beans and coffee may also need to be avoided.

- Colicky babies, for some reason, like their tummies supported. When sitting down, place your infant along your forearm, face down, cradling the head in one hand. This tiger in the tree technique takes practice to perfect.

- Slings are invaluable when your baby is crying inconsolably. Just being nestled against your warm chest is comforting, as is your heartbeat.

- Place your baby in a mechanical baby swing as the continual and steady back-and-forth motion has calmed many distressed babies.

- Get a white or a pink noise app or toy. The sound is like a lullaby to the ears of some colicky infants. Sometimes, colicky babies respond to the sound of a tumble drier, one of ours loved it. Any white or pink noise may work!

- Cut down external stimuli. Sometimes, the more you try to calm a colicky baby, the more he seems to cry. This might be because the baby's nervous system is too immature to handle any noise. Just hold her in your arms and avoid making any noises or eye contact, which is a form of stimulation.

- Do not pat your baby's back when burping her as this can irritate an already-inflamed area. Gently rub in circular motions on the left side of the back or rub upwards with baby's arm straight over your shoulder.

How can paediatric osteopathy benefit babies with lactose overload, colic and gut immaturity?

My view with lactose overload, colic and gut immaturity is that it affects the lower intestinal tract more than any other area of the digestive system. This creates bloating in the large intestine and slows down its peristalsis (wave like muscle contractions that move digested food through the gut). The subsequent explosive poos are the result of large volumes of gas being pushed out. Bloating increases abdominal pressure which gives the baby the typical colic type pain.

Treatment involves releasing tension in the fascial tissue that supports the abdominal organs in order to improve their natural motility (movement). Gentle techniques are applied to synchronise the pump handle and bucket handle action of the ribcage to allow a lengthening of the breathing diaphragm and a deepening of the breath. Pump handle action occurs in the upper ribcage and is an upward movement of the ribs. Bucket handle motion occurs in the lower ribcage and is rib movements to the sides. These are the movements that happen when a child breaths in. This gives the abdominal organs more space to function and enhances digestive clearance.

Olivia's story

Mum brought Olivia to see me at four weeks old. Her birth was eventful, and she was born at 36 weeks by C-section. For the first two weeks Olivia was very good, sleeping well and feeding well on formula. Then Mum noticed a change in Olivia. She was getting trapped wind after drinking her bottles more frequently. Olivia was also grunting and groaning in her sleep especially at night. She was also pushing and straining when trying to do a poo. Bowels were opening with two to four loose motions each day, but Olivia was in pain doing a poo or passing wind. Mum said that Olivia looked bloated.

At night Olivia was restless and grunting throughout the night in her crib. Baby also had a period most nights from 7-9pm where she was crying a lot, going red-faced, looking to feed but refusing, pulling her knees up to her chest and very irritable.

On case history presentation, based on a symptom checklist, my conclusion was that Olivia had colic. My opinion on colic is that it presents as a lower digestive tract problem. Often this is due to wind ingested from a bottle that doesn't suit the baby's sucking action, a formula that is tough on the lower digestive system to digest all day or a gut flora that isn't fully established in young infants.

I treated Olivia's digestive system, focusing on the lower digestive tract. I recommended a change of bottle type, drops to aid lactose digestion and a probiotic for improved gut flora. I gave Mum a Symptom Management Chart to monitor Olivia for the next ten days. Mum returned with baby and reported that her symptoms were significantly better. She had less wind, was pooing easier, had no grunting at night and the evening crying was down to 20–30 minutes, and not every night. Olivia was discharged and check-up booked for one month.

Cow's Milk Protein Allergy

Cow's milk contains two types of protein – whey and casein. Casein is found in the solid part (curd) of milk that curdles. Whey is found in the liquid part of milk that remains after milk curdles.

If your child has a cow's milk protein allergy (CMPA) they may be allergic to only one milk protein or to both. These proteins are hard to avoid because they're also in some processed foods, and most people who react to cow's milk may also react to sheep's, goat's and buffalo's milk. More commonly, people allergic to cow's milk may also be allergic to soya milk. CMPA can be a very complex condition and when we see babies and children who we suspect have a CMPA in our clinic, we always refer them to a paediatric dietician.

CMPA is the most common food allergy seen in infants and children. Between 2% and 7.5% of children are estimated to have CMPA. However, the actual numbers could be much higher as there's a high rate of failure to diagnose the delayed onset type of CMPA. This is backed up by a 2009 study in the UK where it was demonstrated that, of 1000 children with a diagnosis of CMPA, there was considerable under diagnosis, delayed diagnosis and incorrect diagnosis.

CMPA can present with a spectrum of acute or delayed symptoms that can be mild, moderate or severe in nature – easy to see how it can be misdiagnosed or missed, isn't it?

There are two different types of Cows Milk Protein Allergy to look at.

IgE-mediated CMPA – *acute onset*

This type typically occurs within a few minutes of taking cow's milk protein (CMP) and symptoms can range from mild urticaria (rash) to serious anaphylaxis. This is certainly the more serious of the two types and is likely to last longer. It's easier to diagnose as the symptoms relate to the intake of dairy and are obvious. It presents as a very typical allergy that most people will recognise and seek medical attention for.

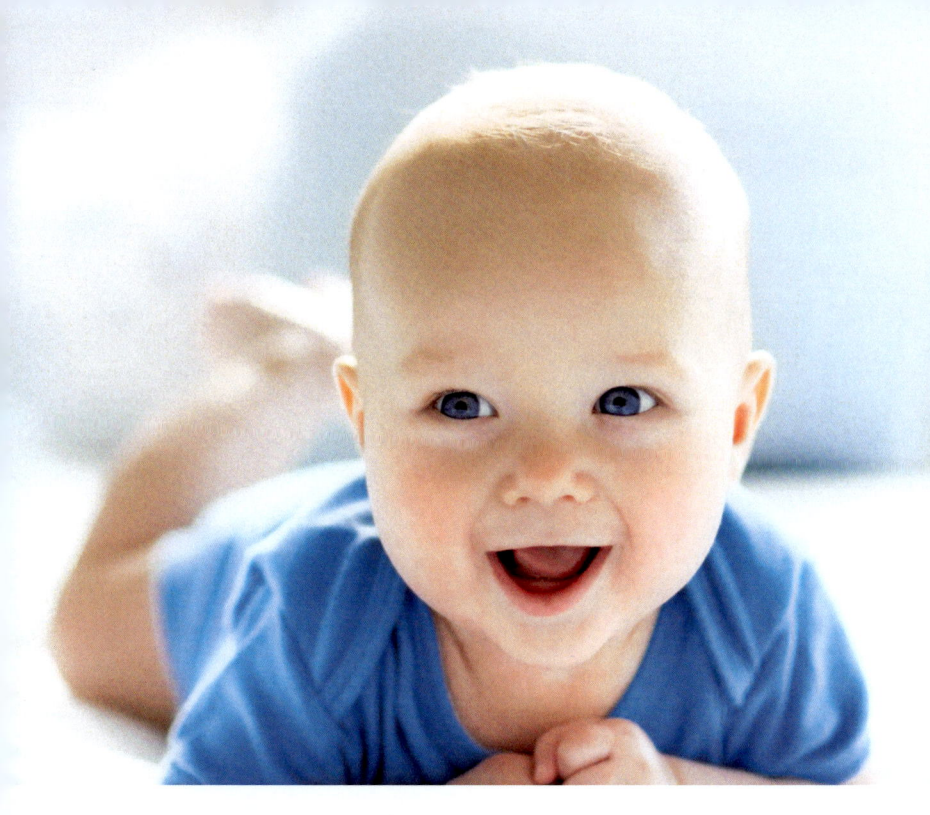

Non IgE-mediated CMPA – *delayed onset*

This type of CMPA occurs several hours or days after taking CMP and tends to affect the gastrointestinal tract, the skin and the respiratory system. This is the type of CMPA we see most frequently at the clinic.

Because of the delayed signs and symptoms, it can be difficult to pinpoint the food causing the allergy in older children and therefore difficult to get a diagnosis. With babies under six months old it's slightly more straightforward as they only drink milk.

There are several circumstances that can help point to a diagnosis of CMPA. Many medical practitioners rely on these associated circumstances to make their diagnosis and therefore it's important to tell your doctor if your baby has any of the following:

- A family history of allergy, most significant in parents and siblings.

- Symptoms that are persistent and affect different systems – gastrointestinal, skin, respiratory.

- Babies who have moderate to severe atopic eczema or dermatitis.
- Babies who have GORD or any other gastrointestinal symptoms such as colic, loose stools or constipation.

Family history of allergy

The results of a 2013 study done in Great Ormond Street Children's Hospital in London demonstrates the importance of a family history of allergy in diagnosing CMPA. The medical notes of 437 children with a confirmed diagnosis of a food protein allergy were looked at. The majority of the children (67.7%) had a family history of allergy. In another study done in 2012 and published in The Journal of Clinical and Diagnostic Research, a family history of allergy was identified in 82.8% of children with CMPA. Interestingly, the most common type of allergic symptoms in a family member were allergic rhinitis (53.8%), food allergy (41.9%), atopic eczema (20.4%) and asthma and respiratory problems (10.8%). For many paediatric dieticians and medical practitioners, a family history of allergy is a very significant fact. While a family history of allergy is important, it's also worth remembering that a lack of family history of allergy does not exclude the possibility of the baby becoming allergic.

General symptoms of CMPA

GASTROINTESTINAL SYMPTOMS
- Vomiting
- Reflux
- Colic
- Diarrhoea
- Constipation
- Flatulence
- Stomach pain
- Mucousy stools
- Distended stomach

ALLERGY CHECKER

SYMPTOM	YOUR CHILD	THE PARENTS	THE SIBLINGS
Eczema			
Hay fever			
Asthma			
Rhinitis			
Food allergy			
Conjunctivitis			
Hives/Rash			

Tick if your child, the parents or the siblings have an allergy

DERMATOLOGICAL SYMPTOMS
- Eczema
- Rashes (skin and nappy)
- Hives (nettle sting type rash)
- Wheals
- Contact dermatitis
- Swelling of the eyes and lips or the whole face or localised swellings (angioedema)

RESPIRATORY SYMPTOMS
- Wheezing
- Sore throat
- Nasal congestion
- Persistent runny nose and/or eyes
- Ear ache
- Persistent cough
- Oral irritation (itchy mouth, excessive dribble)

This list highlights the varying symptoms that may be seen in babies and children with a CMPA and demonstrates the difficulty often experienced in getting a diagnosis.

Symptoms, diagnosis and management of mild to moderate acute onset (IgE-mediated) CMPA

Symptoms of acute onset CMA usually occur within a few minutes and include:

- Skin; acute pruritus (itching), erythema (redness), urticaria (rash like hives), angioedema (swelling). Acute flare up of atopic eczema.
- Gastrointestinal; vomiting, diarrhoea, abdominal pain/colic.
- Respiratory; acute rhinitis and/or conjunctivitis.

Management

If your baby is experiencing severe acute symptoms you should see your doctor.

Although acute onset CMA is less common in breastfed babies, it must be considered if your baby is experiencing some of the above symptoms. Exclusively breastfeeding mothers are advised to remove all dairy from their diet (more information later in the chapter).

Formula-fed babies are changed to an extensively hydrolysed (broken-down) formula and, depending on the results, may need to move to a CMP-free amino acid formula if baby continues to show symptoms of acute CMPA.

A diagnosis is confirmed by a paediatrician by looking at the family history, the reaction of the baby to CMP, the results of a skin prick test or serum IgE test if available and the results of a supervised dairy challenge.

Confirmed cases should always be referred to a paediatric dietician for support and advice about changes in diet and weaning.

Symptoms, diagnosis and management of delayed onset (non IgE-mediated) CMPA

Symptoms of delayed onset CMPA usually occur after several hours or days. Babies can be breastfed, formula-fed or mixed.

- Gastrointestinal: "colic", reflux, food refusal or aversion, loose stools, constipation, abdominal discomfort, blood and/or mucus in stools in an otherwise well baby.
- Skin: Atopic eczema, pruritus.
- Respiratory: cough, nasal congestion

Diagnosis is confirmed only by removing CMP from the diet, the baby improving, and the baby then being challenged with CMP to determine if re-introducing CMP will cause a return of the symptoms.

Management of exclusively breast-fed babies

Exclusively breastfeeding mothers are advised to remove all dairy from their diet. In most cases, symptoms will improve after two to four weeks of an elimination diet. If there is no improvement but allergy is still suspected, then other maternal foods should be considered – e.g. egg, soya. If a breastfeeding mother's diet is to be restricted by more than one food group, it is always wise to consult with a dietician.

If baby's symptoms improve, Mum should avoid CMP until such time as she decides to stop breastfeeding or for at least six months. When Mum decides to stop breastfeeding it's important that a dairy-free amino acid formula is used unless she has done a dairy challenge and has been able to re-introduce dairy back into her diet successfully.

Management of formula fed or mixed feeding babies

If formula fed, change baby to a comfort formula or an extensively hydrolysed formula (EHF). The comfort formula is only suitable for very mild cases of CMPA and for most babies, an EHF is a better option. If you choose a comfort formula and there is no improvement after two weeks, baby should then be changed to an EHF.

Many babies will improve on these formulas but, as there are many levels of sensitivity to CMP, some babies will require a further change to an amino acid formula. These formulas are CMP free.

If mixed feeding, Mum should take all dairy out of her diet and use an EHF for top-ups. Again, if there is no improvement, a further change to an Amino Acid Formula (AAF) may be required or other maternal foods may need to be considered.

What happens next

If your baby has been diagnosed with a CMPA, it is important that CMP is removed from the diet of the baby and/or the breastfeeding mum for at least six months, with the support of a dietician. After six months, your child may be challenged with dairy to see if any symptoms return. For mild to moderate delayed onset CMPA this can usually be done at home. However, for severe delayed onset CMPA and acute onset CMPA this challenge may be better done under the supervision of your dietician or your doctor.

Some babies only present with signs and symptoms of CMPA at weaning. As their dairy intake increases, their intolerance of it reaches tipping point and only then becomes apparent.

Weaning can be a difficult time for CMPA babies as all foods need to be dairy free. Both Nutramigen and Neocate have produced booklets which are available online, to help parents through the choices available. It's also important to be mindful of other new foods introduced in the diet that may pose an allergy risk. The golden rule is to introduce one new food at a time so that if baby reacts to it, it's easily identified! Again, a paediatric dietician will be invaluable during this process.In toddlers, the re-introduction of dairy at home is done using the milk ladder. This is based on the principle that the baking process changes the structure of the milk proteins, thereby making them less allergenic. The interaction between CMP and carbohydrates and fats during the heating process may also reduce the allergenicity of the CMP.

The "milk ladder" is a specific tool used by health professionals and designed for the purpose of creating a tolerance of milk in children who have a milk allergy or a milk sensitivity. To use the milk ladder, most children will start on the bottom step which is the least allergenic. If a step is tolerated, then you should continue to give your child this food while moving up to the next step. How long you stay on each step will be based on the advice of your dietician.

How paediatric osteopathy helps CMPA

When a baby has CMPA their nervous system, in my view, is in "fight or flight" mode. They are in digestive pain, can have reflux, gas, slow bowel clearance and irritation of the skin (eczema). Their body is in distress.

Treatment must focus on calming the nervous system response to distress. Gentle techniques are applied to the cranium to ease muscular tension in the neck. I then work on the respiratory system to ease tension of the ribcage and the breathing diaphragm. This allows decreased traction on the oesophagus as it passes through the breathing diaphragm. This is important for feeding.

I continue with gentle visceral techniques to the abdominal fascia to improve digestive transition in the intestinal tract. Finally, I rebalance the baby's breathing with their cranial motion to establish nervous system calibration.

Removing dairy from your diet if breastfeeding

Breastfeeding is the best milk for your baby. Unfortunately, some proteins in foods you eat can travel through your breast milk to your baby and cause them distress if they have a CMPA. To prevent this from happening, it is important that all cow's milk-based products are removed from your own diet if your health practitioner suspects a CMPA. It is best to also avoid soya products as the incidence of allergy to soya is higher in babies with a CMPA. The incidence of allergy to goat's milk however is less.

Remember also, that CMP can persist in mum's body for one and a half to two weeks, and it may be another one and a half to two weeks before the protein is out of baby's system, so don't expect things to improve dramatically overnight when you make this change. Breastfeeding mums need 1300mgs of calcium in their diet every day so try to use a dairy alternative that is fortified with vitamins and calcium. Otherwise, take a calcium supplement while you are off dairy.

Milk	Almond milk, Koko milk
Yoghurt	Dairy free yoghurt or KoKo yoghurt
Cheese	KoKo dairy free cheese
Cream	Dairy free cream
Ice cream	Dairy free ice cream
Butter	Flora light, olive oil spread

Formulas

Comfort formulas are often a great first step in the treatment of suspected delayed onset CMPA in mild cases. They contain a reduced amount of lactose (the sugar in milk) and partially broken-down CMP.

They can be thicker than a standard formula and may require a change in teat size for comfortable feeding. Try to stay with the brand of formula you are currently using if possible.

Cow & Gate Comfort, SMA Comfort and Aptamil Comfort formulas

These formulas have less than half the lactose of standard baby formulas. They also have partially broken-down (partially hydrolysed) proteins, helping to reduce the potential for feeding discomfort in babies with colic, and contain a special fat blend which helps to produce softer stools. These formulas are also slightly thicker to prevent your baby gulping and taking in too much air during feeding.

EHFs

EHFs are the first choice for babies with moderate delayed onset CMPA and normal growth. The CMP is extensively broken down so that it is more digestible and less allergenic. Whey-based EHFs contain lactose and so are not suitable for babies who have a possible secondary lactose intolerance. Some casein-based formulas are however lactose free and therefore more suitable for these babies.

Many babies have more than one condition. For example, we see many babies who present with reflux and who are later diagnosed with CMPA. Both conditions need to be treated at the same time and this often requires a lot of trial and error. Don't be disheartened though, as there is always a solution.

Aptamil Pepti 1 and Nutramigen Lipil 1 formulas

These are examples of EHFs in which the CMP has been extensively broken down making it easier for babies to tolerate and digest. There can be a taste difference between the regular formulas and these formulas. If baby does not like the new taste, you can blend the new formula with the old formula, slowly increasing the new and decreasing the old formula over a few days. *Aptamil Pepti 1* is a whey-based formula which is suitable for babies from birth. *Nutramigen Lipil 1* is a casein-based formula which is also lactose free. There are other Nutramigen formulas available so it's advisable to consult with your medical practitioner to decide which formula best suits your baby.

AAFs

AAFs are suitable for moderate to severe delayed onset CMPA and all cases of acute onset CMPA. They are CMP free formulas. They are also the formula of choice for exclusively breast-fed babies with a suspected CMA where Mum has eliminated dairy from her diet and the time comes for weaning before a dairy challenge has been done. Examples of AAFs include *Neocate* and *Alfamino*.

Use the chart to document your child's symptoms. When you go to see your health professional, bring your Symptom Checker with you as this will be helpful in assisting them to make a diagnosis. It also ensures that you will remember to tell your health professional everything.

CMPA SYMPTOM CHECKER

Vomiting	Wheals
Reflux	Contact dermatitis
Colic	Swelling of the eyes, lips, face
Diarrhoea	
Constipation	Severe pruritus
Flatulence	Wheezing
Mucus in the stools	Sore throat
Blood in the stools	Persistent runny nose/ eyes
Stomach pain/discomfort	Itchy mouth or excessive dribble
Distended stomach	
Food aversion or refusal	Acute rhinitis
Eczema	Conjunctivitis
Rashes-skin or nappy	Nasal congestion
Hives	

Tick if your baby has this symptom

At the back of this book you will find a Symptom Management Chart. By observing and grading five key areas you will get a broad picture of how baby is doing over a full week. This allows you to record the various symptoms to allow your medical practitioner to look at them objectively.

Both this chart and the Symptom Management Chart are available to download free from our website.

Paul's story

Mum brought Paul to see me when he was twelve weeks old. He was born at 39 weeks following an eight hour labour which was uneventful. Mum described Paul as irritable in general with a very poor sleeping pattern. Paul had difficulties feeding and taking all his feeds, burping was tough and his bowels were very variable as he might not poo for four to five days.

Mum had changed formula four times from the standard formula to a comfort formula to lactose free formula and finally returned to a standard formula again. She said there was very little difference in him when formulas were changed. Paul had recently developed nasal congestion and
was now wheezing. Mum had taken Paul to the doctor to check his chest which was clear.

He had also developed a rash on his face, eyebrows and scalp which would ease when a cream was applied but would return after stopping the application of the cream. His skin had a dry appearance and was starting to look redder in recent weeks.

On case history examination, I was particularly interested in the family history of food allergies, asthma, hay fever and eczema. Mum stated that dad had eczema as a young baby, cried for nine months and was put on goat's milk formula. Paul's brother, who was now three years old, had chronic reflux as a baby and developed asthma as a toddler. Mum said they changed formulas for his reflux numerous times but that he just "grew out of it" at ten months. "He still doesn't like milk and prefers drinking water," she added.

My view on this case was that Paul could have a CMPA. I treated Paul's digestive system to give him ease and referred him to a paediatric dietician to establish if he had CMPA. The dietician switched Paul to a specific formula for CMPA and would review him in a month.

I saw Paul at the clinic five weeks later. His skin condition had cleared up. He didn't have a wheeze, he was pooing most days and his Mum reported that he was less irritable and was sleeping much better.

The key to this case is the presenting symptoms and family history. You must be objective in considering the presenting symptoms and be open-minded. Not every presentation is colic or reflux. Look at the details. CMPA is often a slow onset condition and it can take a while for the symptoms to develop. They can develop in three systems, digestive, respiratory and skin. It is important to refer to a paediatrician or paediatric dietician in these cases, to seek their expert opinion.

Paul was assisted with weaning by the paediatric dietician and was later guided back onto diary using the milk ladder under the supervision of the dietician.

Sleep

To most new parents sleep is priceless! But to be fair, when a new baby arrives it is expected that sleep will not be something you will be getting too much of for the next little while. Sleep can become the most valuable commodity in your home, and you may find yourself comparing who got how many hours sleep last night. I know we did.

However, when baby becomes a toddler and the months drag on with no end or sleep in sight, it is normal for parents to look for a solution. Many parents will have tried some form of sleep training without success before they come to us. The way we have always approached sleep is to look for a possible physical reason to explain why little one's sleep is disturbed. Finding and treating this is usually the answer. When no physical issue is found, it allows parents to start sleep training with confidence.

"People who say they sleep like a baby usually don't have one."

What is normal for your baby?

Newborn babies sleep a lot, typically about eight to eighteen hours a day. But they sleep in short cycles so, to many new parents, it may feel like they never sleep. The circadian rhythms, which are regulated by light and dark, can take time to develop, explaining the irregular sleep schedules of new-borns. Small babies also have small tummies and need to wake frequently to feed. The sleep/wake cycles begin to develop at about six weeks, and by three to six months most babies begin to sleep for longer stretches during the night and are more wakeful during the day.

A baby's sleep cycle is different from that of an adult. It is shorter, lasting between 50-60 minutes or less. Sleep is divided into 50% active (REM) sleep and 50% quiet (non-REM) sleep. During active sleep a baby is more likely to wake up. They take shallow breaths and twitch their arms and legs. Their eyes can flutter under their eyelids. About halfway through a sleep cycle, your baby will change to quiet sleep. Their breathing will become slower and more rhythmic. They will move less and there will be no eyelid fluttering. After quiet sleep, your baby will either wake up or return to active sleep.

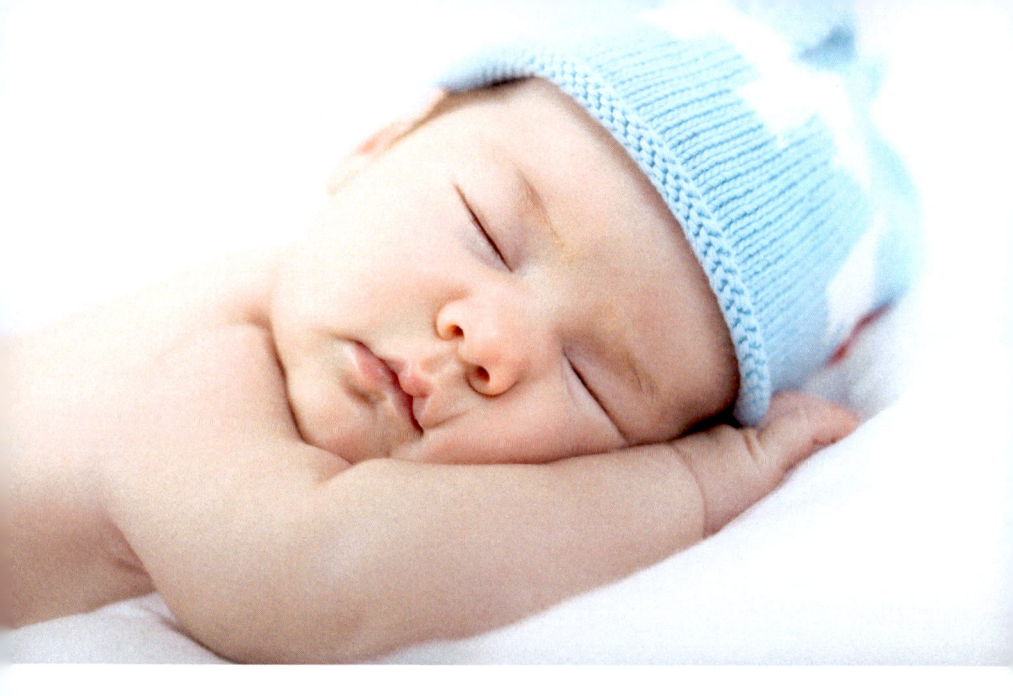

Sleep is important for your child in the early months and years. It assists brain development. Babies need sleep so that they can assimilate everything they have learned and experienced. Blood flow to the brain nearly doubles during active sleep. When a baby's brain is growing and developing the most is also the time when they have more active sleep. Premature babies spend even more of their sleep-time in active sleep, perhaps up to 90%. As baby gets older active sleep comprises about 30% of sleep.

From three to six months, most babies begin to settle into a better sleep pattern. They are more wakeful for longer stretches during the day and may sleep for up to five to eight hours at a time at night. Between three to six months, they can continue to wake once or twice for feeds at night.

After six months you will notice that they now have less active sleep and more quiet sleep. Managing the night-time waking is important now as baby has learned new skills. They acquire the ability to stay awake while at the same time they are learning new exciting skills such as sitting up and crawling. This combination of being able to do exciting new things and being able to stay awake can mean your baby might wake more often during the night and be more reluctant to go back to sleep. They also figure out object permanence. This is the ability to understand that an object can exist even if they cannot see it. As a result of this, when they do wake at night, they may call out for you.

How to recognise sleep cues

Most babies will follow a reasonably predictable pattern with regards to sleep but it's worth being aware of the subtle hints your baby will give you when they are ready for a sleep.

- Yawning
- Frowning
- Decreased activity
- Less vocal and interactive
- Sucking is weaker or slower
- Quieter and calmer
- Eyes less focused
- Rubbing eyes or ears
- Eyes closing down
- Fussiness
- Hard to distract and keep happy

What can stop your little one from sleeping through the night?

The first thing to look at is conditioning or habit. Has your child become accustomed to waking up for a feed, a chat and a cuddle at night? Do they come into your bed most nights? Do they need you with them to fall asleep? It's always a good idea to set the night-time ground rules as early as possible. Night-time should be quiet. The room should remain as dark as possible so that there's a big difference between day and night. If you turn on the lights and chat and do all the things you would do during the day, how will baby be able to tell the difference?

With a toddler who may have acquired a few bad habits, the first step is to establish a good bedtime routine. Set a time each evening when this starts and stick to it every night. Start with bath-time, followed by cuddles and a feed if they still require one. Then read them a bed-time story in their room. Finally, settle them down and leave the room. It will take a little while for this new routine to be totally adopted with as much enthusiasm as you have for it, but it will happen. Just be patient and give it time.

Ensure that the new routine is followed by anyone who puts baby to bed. Consistency is key here. There are so many good books on the market describing different methods of sleep training. Feel free to select the one that suits you and your family best. The book we recommend is *The Baby Sleep Solution* by Lucy Wolfe. Lucy's approach is a gentle supportive one and she has had amazing success with it.

For children who have persistent colds and coughs, nasal drip could be an issue and a cause of sleep disruption. Children who have a nasal drip affecting the respiratory passages are often congested and frequently have a runny nose. They can be mouth breathers and as a result snore at night. This too can disrupt their sleep and wake them up.

The other type of nasal drip is a posterior nasal drip, and, in this case, the drip affects the back of the throat and the Eustachian tubes (narrow tubes connecting the middle ear to the back of the throat) causing a cough and congestion. There can be nasal congestion with this type too. These symptoms can disrupt the child's sleep.

Children who have had ear infections may have some fluid in the middle ear and this too can disrupt sleep. Cranial osteopathy is used here to release any tension in the bones of the skull, particularly the temporal bones which house the middle and inner ears. A product we also recommend for children with nasal congestion is a salt pump.

Used at night in the room the child sleeps in, it can help clear out the mucus and aid a good night's sleep.

Salin Salt Pump – This great little salt pump gives you all the benefits of salt therapy but at home. It works by pushing the air through a filter which contains a micro-crystallised deposit of salts, primarily sodium chloride – 98% NaCl, 0.5% calcium chloride and magnesium, 0.2% iodine and sulphur. Use is recommended mainly at night to ensure minimum exposure of eight hours a day. If necessary, exposure can be extended to the whole day. The feedback we have received from parents of children with congestion has been very positive and it continues to be a product we recommend very frequently.

Vicks Warm Mist Humidifier – This is another great product for children with coughs, colds and congestion. You could also add a few drops of Olbas Oil to the humidifier to help a blocked nose. Ideal for helping little one get a little sleep!

Another reason for sleep disruption is a digestive disorder. Reflux, wind or allergy can cause enough discomfort at night to wake baby. Again, cranial osteopathy can help relieve these issues, along with advice depending on which condition is affecting baby. Once any cranial and physical issues are dealt with, baby should be able to develop a better sleeping pattern with a little help from Mum and Dad (see tips below). There can be other less common issues but, in our experience, these are the main reasons for a disturbed sleep pattern in young children. So, if you are having difficulties with your toddler maybe you should consider the above as possible causes. Remember, it's always wise to rule out any physical issue before you start sleep training. There is always a solution and every child will learn to sleep through the night. It may require patience, persistence and perhaps a little cranial osteopathy but you will get there in the end!

Top tips for sleep

Establishing good sleep routines from the start will pay dividends in the long run. It will take a few months for baby to settle into what you could loosely describe as a routine. The sleep hormone melatonin isn't fully produced by infants until almost twelve weeks, which means they don't have a proper "schedule" until then. But if you do the ground work early you will sow the seeds of a great sleep-time schedule.

A baby's sleep cycle is shorter than an adult, at about 45–60 minutes. If your baby wakes up after this length of time, try being extra quiet as they transition from one sleep cycle to another. A baby can take as long as twenty minutes to reach a deep sleep. If baby wakes after a short while, they may not have reached deep sleep. Try to settle them down again or if a little older, leave to settle themselves back to sleep.Sleeping through the night is generally described as baby getting seven to twelve consecutive hours of sleep, which to be honest, is a dream come true for any new parent. One of the best ways to achieve this is a good bedtime routine. There are many different methods of sleep training but the common thread to success with all of them is consistency. Everyone putting baby to sleep must follow the same routine. Decide on a plan and stick to it. Agree with your partner about who'll do what when baby wakes.

Before you start sleep training, it is always best to rule out any physical issues that may be interrupting your baby's sleep.

Creating consistent routines for your baby will help bring order to what can be a very chaotic world. A bedtime routine may consist of a bath, a massage, a story, a feed and off to sleep. Keep the room dim and as the routine progresses, soften your voice and talk less. Have a few phrases that you repeat such as "night, night, we love you" or "sleepy time now" – whatever works for you. Have a routine for daytime naps too. This can be shorter but will have similar elements.

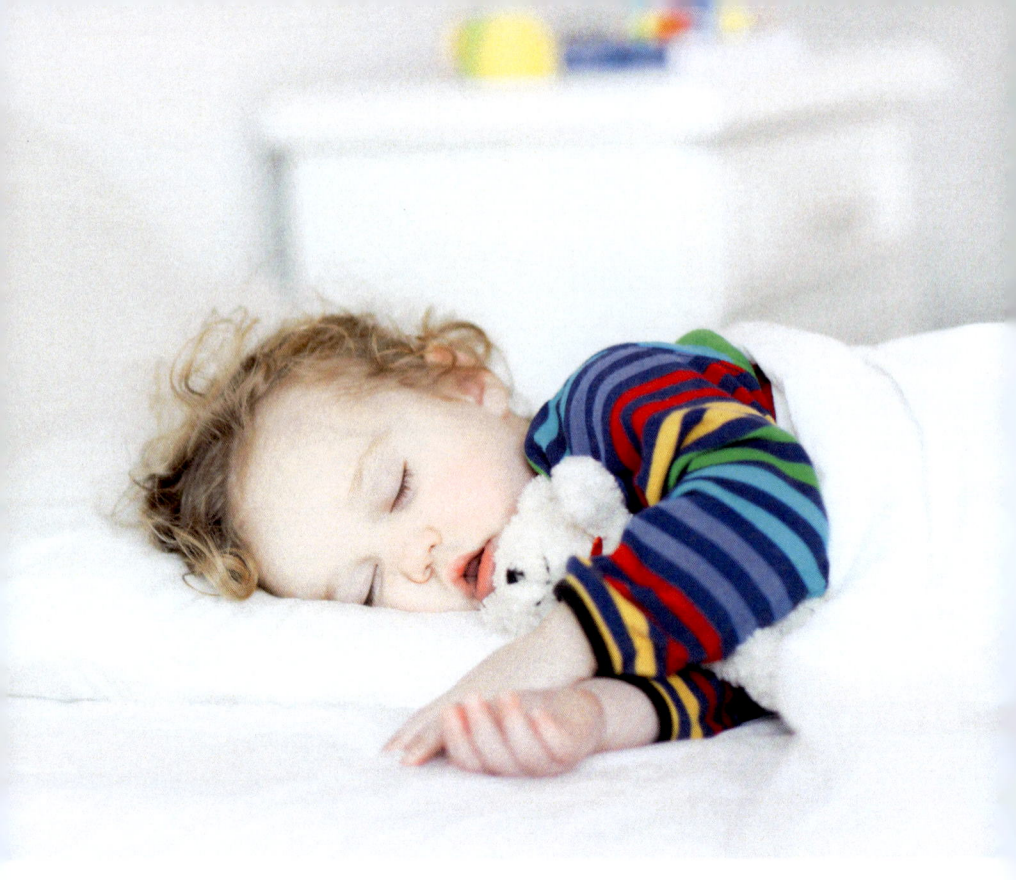

It may include closing the curtains, placing baby in his crib, cuddles and a few sleepy phrases such as "sleep well, we love you".

A dreamfeed is something that can work for some babies. This is a feed just before you go to bed yourself. Baby is sleeping but you gently lift them from their crib and give a sleeping feed. Once they have fed, settle them down gently again. It's a great way to ensure that Mum gets a little sleep at night and works well for the first few months.

As tempting as it is to leave a sleeping baby sleep on, when it comes to daytime naps, this is not advised. The longer a baby sleeps during the day, the more likely it is to affect night-time sleep. Of course, as children get a little older, there will be times when they will need a long recovery nap – a very busy day or a poor sleep the night before perhaps. Keep watch on how long baby is napping for and don't be afraid to wake them if it extends past two and a half hours.

White or pink noise is a very popular way of ensuring baby gets a better sleep. Before birth, baby was exposed to white sounds and Mum's heartbeat. Using white or pink noise in the early days can be a very soothing way to comfort baby. You can get a phone app, buy a small device or simply turn on the dryer or a fan. You don't need to have it at full volume though, a low volume near baby will work just fine. White noise in the form of a dryer was a godsend for one of our girls. It cancelled out all the normal house noises allowing her to sleep in peace. She is using white noise again now as she studies for her Leaving Certificate Examination!

Another long-established sleep training tool is the eat, wake, sleep cycle. This method is very useful for younger babies but can be used for babies until they are completely weaned off formula or breast milk. When baby wakes in the morning, or after a nap, they are fed immediately. This will mean that baby is most alert when feeding and will be more likely to take more. It also means that baby will not associate a feed with sleep and will be better at self-soothing. Having said this, there will be times when your little one will need a feed before sleep and that's fine. It's not a rule to set in stone, rather a suggestion to use when it suits your baby. Of course, newborn babies will not fall into this cycle as they will require more frequent feeding and will sleep more too.

In our opinion, nappy changes at night are on an only if needed basis. A good quality absorbent nappy should see baby through the night. A quick sniff test will let you know if it should be changed. If a change is needed, a quick quiet one is best. Avoid the chatter as you want baby to remember it's night-time. You could probably do a nappy change with your eyes closed by that stage so minimal lighting is all that's required. If baby has a skin irritation or nappy rash, then the change will be needed.

If baby wakes in the night-time, don't rush in straight away. Baby may self-sooth and go back to sleep. This is a very valuable skill to learn and you rushing in at the first movement will only delay its learning. Sometimes baby will cry briefly or babble and if baby does not settle, then get to him before he is too woken up and less likely to go back to sleep. Ideally, it's best to put baby down to sleep when awake but drowsy. This also teaches them the skill of self-soothing. Babies, like adults, will naturally wake up during the night as they transition from one sleep cycle to the next. Without knowing how to get back to sleep, a baby will cry out after waking. As baby gets older, being able to fall asleep independently allows them to drift back to sleep after waking in the night, helping baby sleep better in the long run.

Eye contact with your baby is wonderful. His heart rate increases, his blood pressure rises and he becomes more awake. So, you can see that eye contact in the middle of the night will have the opposite effect to what you want. Instead, keep your gaze on his tummy and rub his back to sooth him. Keeping interactions with your little one to a minimum can be difficult but by doing so, it re-enforces the day-time and night-time differences. Do have plenty of eye contact with your baby the next morning as it boosts brain development and bonding and signals it's daytime. Likewise, chatting to baby will stimulate brain activity as babies are programmed to react to their mother's voice.

Incorporating baby massage into your night-time sleep routine is a wonderful way to relax baby. Some gentle and soothing music and a warm comfortable environment will add to the benefits. Studies have shown that babies who had a bedtime massage fell asleep faster and slept more soundly than those who didn't have one. As you massage baby, slow down your own breathing. This sends a signal to baby to be calm.

There will be times when sleep goes out the window, but don't panic. It's probably just a minor upset, and things will soon settle down again. Babies and toddlers can often have sleep regressions around major developmental milestones or when they are sick or when routines at home change. A new baby, holidays or Christmas can all upset their routine and once you keep consistent about what you can control, things will improve again in time.

How paediatric osteopathy can help sleep

There may be physical signs why your baby or child wakes up during the night and has a broken sleep pattern. It is important to check respiratory and digestive function. Disruption to these systems in my view, creates over-stimulation of the nervous system which in turn affects sleep.

Treatment should focus on gentle techniques to the cranial base muscularly to enhance mucous drainage. Treatment opens up the ribcage motion by releasing intercostal muscle tension. This establishes a deeper breathing pattern. I improve visceral organ clearance by lengthening fascial tissue supporting the organs in position. Finally, I ease the occiput-sacral tension by gentle techniques which balance the skeletal system.

Grace's story

Mum brought Grace to the clinic when she was nine months old. Mum said that Grace had been waking four to five times a night, usually distressed and crying, wanting to be picked up and either fed or rocked back to sleep. I found it interesting that Mum said at times, Grace would not want to take a feed and would refuse it. Grace was a formula fed baby.

On questioning Mum about Grace, she said that Grace had a good night-time routine. It started at 7.30pm with a bath, then she got dressed into night clothes, was given a bottle feed and read a story. After this she was placed into her crib with Mum sitting beside Grace, which allowed her to go off to sleep in a gentle self-soothing way. Grace would sleep well until after 1am and then would repeatedly wake up.

Grace also had a good daytime nap routine. She would sleep for 60 minutes in the morning usually between 9–10am. Again, she had a nap in the afternoon from 1.30–2.30pm and a brief siesta from 5–5.45pm. This helped Grace rest and not get over-tired.

When questioning Mum, I wanted to know if there was any underlying physical condition that had been troubling Grace. Mum stated that Grace had colic from weeks three to eight and this had then settled down. She had been teething from month four and had been generally ok with this. At month six she had developed a bronchiolitis from a virus – she was seen by her GP.

After the virus Grace had continued to have congestion that wasn't clearing. She also had a mucous cough from time to time, runny nose and a mild wheeze that came and went. When I asked Mum about her sleeping pattern, she said that Grace was very restless before she first woke up, pulling at her ears and rolling her head on the mattress. She would sit up and then begin crying. Mum had taken Grace to her doctor who checked the chest and ears. They were all clear.

On examination, I found that Grace had a mild bronchial wheeze and her upper ribcage had tension muscularly in the pump handle movement. The key finding was when I palpated behind her ears and gently tugged on the earlobe. Grace was very sensitive to touch in this area. My view was she had developed glue ear. This is a condition in which fluid is trapped behind the eardrum and this can cause increased pressure especially when you lie down, like the feeling that you can get on a plane coming into land – a fullness in the ear.

This condition affects some toddlers and, in my opinion can disturb sleep patterns. I treated Grace at the clinic to assist the drainage of the ear and improve overall rib action. I also advised Mum to get a decongestion pump to help clear the mucous at night. I asked Mum to return in a week to check if the sleep pattern had changed.

When I saw Grace ten days later, she looked rested. Mum said that as the time went on Grace was sleeping for longer periods at night, her cough had subsided, runny nose was less evident, and pulling at her ears had stopped. She was more restful when asleep. Her physical condition had been impacting on her sleep pattern. This is an important finding and, in my opinion, should always be checked before sleep training commences.

Tongue-tie

Most of us think of tongue-tie as a situation we find ourselves in when we are too excited to speak. But tongue-tie is the non-medical term for a relatively common but often overlooked physical condition, that limits the use of the tongue.

Tongue-tie affects 5–10% of newborn babies and is more common in boys than girls. Normally, the tongue is loosely attached to the base of the mouth with a piece of skin called the lingual frenulum. In babies with tongue-tie, this piece of skin is unusually short and tight, restricting the tongue's movement. The medical name for tongue-tie is ankyloglossia. Tongue-tie can run in families, with some only mildly affected, and others whose function is severely affected.

For some babies, tongue-tie will be almost unnoticeable. They will feed normally and as they grow the frenulum will stretch and loosen so that their speech will not be affected. For other babies, tongue-tie will be a problem, particularly when it comes to feeding. Not all tongue-ties look the same, making diagnosis difficult at times.

The biggest effect of a tongue-tie in a newborn baby, is on the breastfeeding baby. To breastfeed successfully, the baby needs to latch on to both breast tissue and nipple, and the baby's tongue needs to cover the lower gum, so the nipple is protected from damage. Babies with tongue-tie are not able to open their mouths wide enough to latch on to their mother's breast properly. They tend to slide off the breast and grind on the nipple with their gums. This is very painful, and the mother's nipples can become sore. Some babies feed poorly and get tired, but they soon become hungry and want to feed again.

Many mums experiencing this type of difficulty with breastfeeding will look for advice from a lactation consultant. Tongue-tie should always be out ruled or diagnosed by a health professional in breastfeeding mums who are having feeding difficulties.

Tongue-tie is more common in boys than girls.

Of course, bottle-fed babies can also have a tongue-tie. While feeding is less dependent on the good movement of the tongue, very often these babies can take in a lot of air when feeding. They can gulp their feed and will be on and off the teat often during the feed. We often see babies who have symptoms very similar to reflux as a result of tongue-tie. For this reason, it is always worthwhile checking for the possibility of tongue- or lip-tie in babies with reflux symptoms.

Symptoms of tongue-tie

SYMPTOMS MAY INCLUDE:

- Falls asleep while feeding
- Poor latch
- Slides off nipple during feeds
- Audible clicking noise while feeding
- Reflux symptoms
- Poor weight gain
- Gumming/chewing of Mum's nipples while feeding
- Short sleep episodes requiring feeds every two to three hours
- When baby cries the tongue can be seen to be suspended in the mouth with the sides curled upwards at the edges.

MUM'S SIGNS AND SYMPTOMS MAY INCLUDE:

- Cracked, bruised and blistered nipples
- Creased, flattened or blanched nipples after breastfeeding
- Bleeding nipples
- Severe pain when baby attempts to latch
- Poor or incomplete breast drainage
- Mastitis or nipple thrush
- Plugged ducts

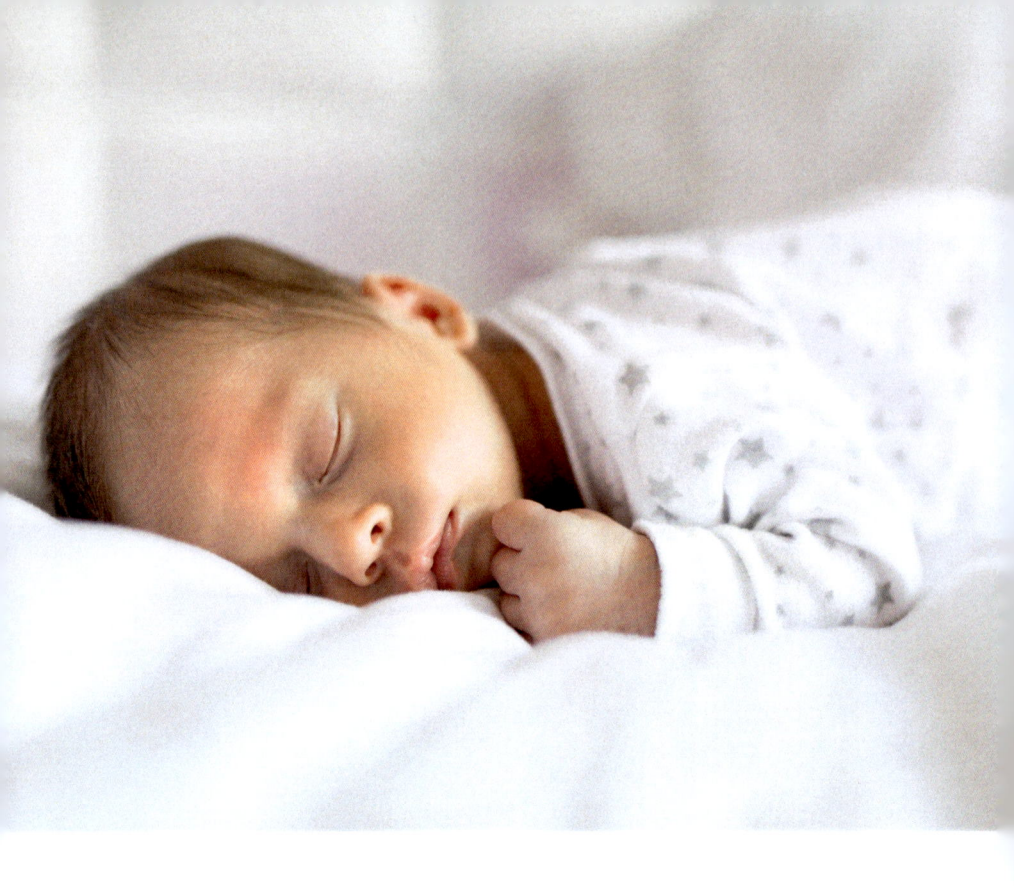

In many cases, these feeding difficulties mean the baby fails to gain enough weight. Although it is often overlooked, tongue-tie can be an underlying cause of feeding problems that not only affect a child's weight gain but lead many mothers to abandon breastfeeding altogether.

Lip-tie

A lip-tie is very similar to a tongue-tie. With a lip-tie, the piece of tissue connecting the upper lip to the gum is too tight. This prevents the upper lip from flaring out and creating a good seal on the breast. In some cases, a baby may even have difficulty feeding from a bottle. Treatment for a lip-tie is to release it by cutting the frenulum connecting the upper lip to the gum. Many children who have a lip-tie can also have a tongue-tie. Both can be released at the same time.

How to correct tongue-tie

Once a tongue-tie has been diagnosed by your lactation consultant, osteopath or doctor, it's then time to get treatment. Every area has a specialised dentist, GP or paediatrician who performs a procedure called a frenotomy.

A frenotomy is a surgical incision of the lingual frenulum, the band of tissue that connects the base of the tongue to the floor of the mouth. It is done with a sterile scissors or by laser.

In older children, a mild general anaesthetic may be given, while a local anaesthetic gel is applied to the area under the tongue in babies. Most babies will cry a little during the procedure due to the lifting up of the tongue to access the area. The procedure takes as little as one minute. Once the frenotomy is done, baby can breastfeed immediately.

Very often, a lactation consultant will see you after the procedure to advise you about feeding positions and to ensure that baby is now feeding better than before the procedure. You will be advised about pain relief for your baby as it is very important to keep baby comfortable while the wound is healing so that they can tolerate the mouth work required and that they will continue to feed and move their tongue.

You will be given very specific exercises to do with baby to prevent the tongue-tie re-occurring. When doing these exercises, it's very important to pick a time of day when baby is most settled and has had pain relief. For a small baby, mid-feed is a good time.

Possible effects of an untreated tongue-tie

Very often, a tongue-tie will remain undiagnosed, and it's not until the child is older and presents with other issues that it comes to light. Sometimes, parents decide to stop breastfeeding in order to resolve the feeding issues occurring as a result of a tongue-tie. While this may solve the immediate feeding issue, it may be storing other problems for later.

We have seen babies at seven or eight months who require frenotomy as they are having difficulty eating solids. They cannot move their tongue sufficiently to manoeuvre the food to swallow it and often they just spit it back out. They regularly gag and choke on food and are persistent dribblers. These children can become picky eaters as they prefer softer food and tend to not eat age-appropriate foods.

As the child gets older, they may have speech difficulties. The tongue is a vital part in speech development and any restriction of it may have a negative impact on speech. Having a tongue-tie will also put the older child at risk of needing orthodontic treatment to straighten teeth.

It's vital to do the post-frenotomy exercises regularly, even if they cause a little upset for baby. It will be worth it in the end.

How paediatric osteopathy can help tongue-tie

I will often see babies when they have had a frenotomy (tongue-tie correction) done. The key to treatment is the re-balancing of muscular tension in the front and the back of the neck. Prior to having the frenotomy, the baby's tongue has been anchored to the floor of the mouth and unable to form a good latch. The neck and jaw muscles have been used to create the latch and that becomes exhausting for the baby when feeding.

Once the tongue-tie is released the baby will learn to orientate the movement of the tongue to deepen the latch. I use very gentle techniques to ease tension in the muscles of the neck and the jaw to allow the baby's latch to improve. Re-balancing of the neck muscles will allow the baby to rotate to both sides more easily and have the head in a neutral position for feeding.

Improving ribcage movement allows an improved suck-breath-swallow mechanism to occur when baby is feeding.

Padraig's story

Mum brought Padraig to the clinic when he was five weeks old. Mum was exclusively breast feeding and was encountering difficulties with Padraig when feeding him. She said several signs were present, short feeds, falling asleep when feeding, clicking when feeding, having to re-latch when feeding, sore, cracked nipples which were now recovering, spitting up breast milk, feeding every two hours most of the day and stretching to three to four hours at night. Mum said Padraig appeared to be in pain after spitting up and looked to feed almost immediately again as if to soothe the discomfort.

Mum had gone to her breastfeeding group and got great advice from the nurses to allow her to continue breastfeeding. However Mum said that feeding was becoming more demanding as Padraig was getting older.

I examined Padraig and noticed immediately that his musculature was in high tension at the back of his neck. When

he cried his tongue was suspended in the mid mouth, curling up on both sides with a depression in the mid tongue area. When I tested his sucking reflex, he was engaging his jaw to create suction and his upper lip turned downwards to latch. The sucking action was weak, and he was taking a lot of air in as he continued sucking.

My view was that he had a possible tongue-tie and lip-tie. I advised Mum to get this checked by a lactation consultant nurse colleague of mine, who confirmed the diagnosis and referred Padraig to a paediatrician who treated the tongue-tie (frenotomy).

Padraig returned fourteen days later to the clinic. Mum said his feeding pattern had greatly improved, longer feeds, deeper latch, less spitting up, improved sleep pattern and altogether a happier, more contented baby. I treated the muscular areas of the neck to ease any tension post tongue-tie to improve Padraig's head position when feeding.

The key finding here is that feeding is a mechanical action that requires total coordination. If the action of the tongue is impeded, the baby will adapt but will struggle to achieve good control of the feeding action.

Plagiocephaly

In the 1990's, following on from very conclusive research, doctors started recommending that all babies be put to sleep on their backs to reduce the risk of sudden infant death syndrome (SIDS) or cot death. Since the start of this campaign, the incidence of SIDS has dropped by almost 40%. This was a major discovery and since then the advice has been that babies should sleep on their backs. However, the slight downside of this is that there has been a related increase in the number of children who have developed positional plagiocephaly (or positional flat head syndrome).

A study done in 2014 in Canada looked at the incidence of positional plagiocephaly in a group of full-term infants who attended for their two month check at four different well-child clinics. The results were startling. The incidence of positional plagiocephaly was estimated to be 46.6%. The identified risk factors included having a right or left sided head position preference, having had a vacuum or forceps assisted delivery and being male. Thankfully, this is a minor condition, that if diagnosed and treated early, can be resolved very easily.

What is positional plagiocephaly?

Plagiocephaly is a condition where the back or side of the baby's head appears to be flattened. It can be congenital (present at birth) or it can develop during infancy (positional). Congenital plagiocephaly is caused by a relatively rare condition called craniosynostosis where the bones of the skull fuse too soon.

Positional plagiocephaly is caused by environmental factors, delivery factors or by the baby resting its head for long periods against flat surfaces, including car seats or cot mattresses. Because babies' skulls are made up of several different plates that are not yet fused together, they are much more susceptible to external pressures and are therefore prone to the condition.

Plagiocephaly occurs either evenly across the back of the head, or off to one side. This is because some babies lie with their head straight while others prefer it turned.

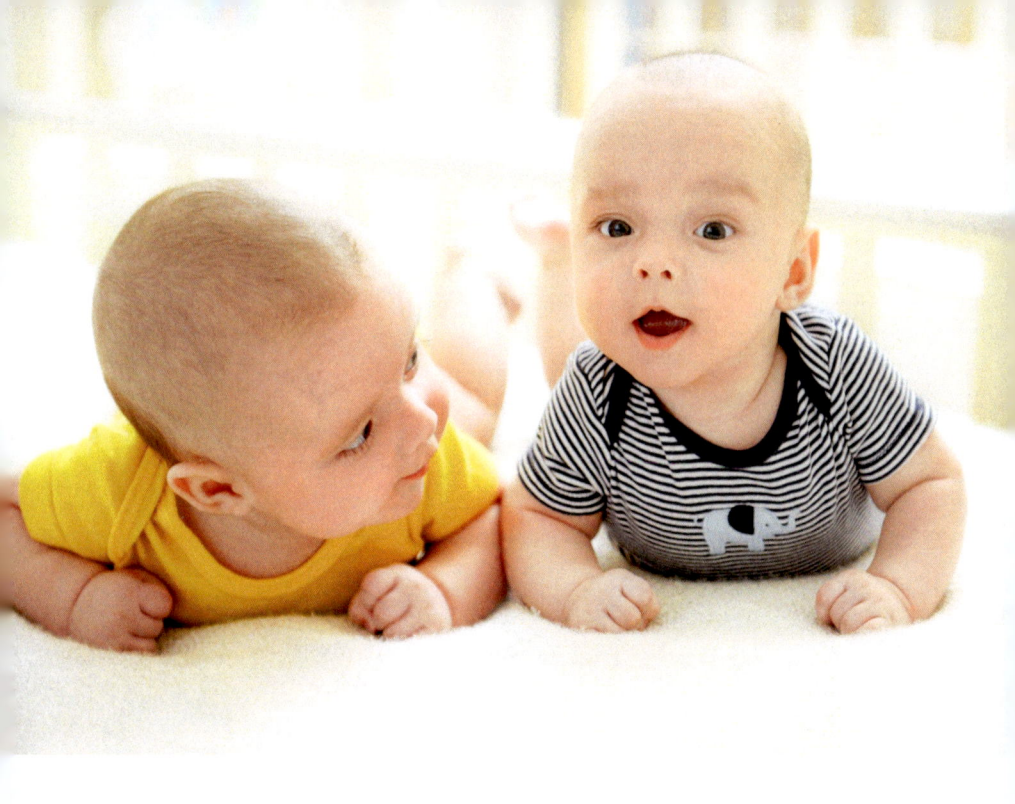

Positional plagiocephaly can also occur in babies with shortened or tightened neck muscles on one side. This prevents baby's head from turning freely and is known as Congenital Torticollis. Positional Plagiocephaly can also develop before a baby is even born if pressure is placed on his skull by the mother's pelvis or from a twin.

Premature infants are more prone to developing positional plagiocephaly because their skulls are softer and more pliant, and because they tend to spend a greater amount of time on their backs. Babies born by vacuum or forceps delivery are also at risk due to the overstretching of the neck muscles during delivery.

Whatever the cause, rest assured plagiocephaly is quite common and it's not your fault. While it can be very unsettling for some parents to see the shape of their baby's head has altered, for most babies it's a condition that can be very easily treated. And certainly the sooner treatment starts the better the success rate.

> *As soon as you notice that your baby turns their head to one side more than the other, you should see your health practitioner. The sooner treatment starts, the better for baby.*

Torticollis

Congenital torticollis is present at birth. It's a condition where the neck muscles on one side are tighter and therefore shorter than the other side. This results in baby tilting and/or turning their head to one side predominantly. If it were you or I, we would be stretching our tight neck, but a baby just stays with what is most comfortable for them.

The main causes of congenital torticollis are an instrumental delivery and breech delivery. In both cases, the sternomastoid muscle (the muscle that extends from the jaw to the collarbone and breastbone) is overstretched.

Plagiocephaly risk factors

- Baby who spends too much time lying on their back in car seats or cots. It's still recommended however, that babies sleep on their backs as the benefit of reducing SIDS far outweighs any dangers due to positional plagiocephaly.
- Twin pregnancy/Multiple birth.
- Prematurity.
- Instrumental delivery – vacuum or forceps.
- Long labour.

How is positional plagiocephaly detected?

Typically, parents notice that their baby's head is flattened at the back or on one side. It is not painful and does not affect the baby's everyday life or his abilities. The following could be signs of head flattening:

- head turned one way most of the time
- flat spot on back or one side of the head
- one ear more forward than the other
- asymmetry of the face

Treatment

Most of a child's skull growth occurs during infancy. The sooner plagiocephaly is diagnosed and treatment is started, the better. Most treatment options centre around tummy time, adding in specific exercises in more ongoing cases. In this instance, the support of a paediatric physiotherapist will be invaluable.

Skull growth slows, and the skull hardens during the toddler years. Early prevention and treatment are therefore important. Below are examples of ways you can improve head flattening and your child's neck mobility.

- Minimise use of or time spent in car seats and baby carriers – these cause a constant pressure to the back of the head. Many These inserts offer support and create a softer resting surface for the head.
- Use a Baby Pillow specifically for plagiocephaly such as the *Mimos* pillow.
- Ensure toys and communication are to the non-affected side to encourage baby to look away from the flattened side. This applies to toys attached to the side of the cot as well as play during the daytime.
- Change the arm or hip you carry your baby on to encourage him to turn his head away from the flattened side.

- When feeding, hold your baby so that he must turn his head away from the side of the flattening to feed. This may take a little time for baby to be happy about, but persistence will pay off. If your child is a little older and in a high chair, feed them from the opposite side to the flattening.

- During a nappy change, work again at the non-affected side to encourage baby to turn his head to this side and away from the flattened side.

- When your baby is alert (after a night's sleep or nap time), provide plenty of supervised 'tummy time'. This is a great way to avoid pressure on the back of the head but is also an excellent developmental exercise to help improve head and neck control.

Mimos plagiocephaly pillow

We have been recommending the *Mimos pillow* for a while now and the feedback from parents has been amazing. The difference in the shape of baby's head, even after two weeks, has been very encouraging. The sooner you start using the pillow the better the results as the bones of the skull have less movement as baby gets older.

The Mimos pillow was designed specially to prevent and correct cranial deformities during baby's first few months. The pillow increases the area of contact beneath the head thereby reducing the pressure by up to four times. It comes in a few sizes depending on the circumference of baby's head. It's breathable and washable. It is an investment well worth making as the results speak for themselves.

Tummy time

Because tummy time relieves pressure from the back of a baby's head, it is an excellent way to prevent and treat head flattening. This is also a great position for strengthening the head and neck muscles. The muscles that extend the neck and keep the head up against gravity, are attached at the base of the skull at the back. When a baby is on its tummy, these muscles contract and work hard to keep the head up.

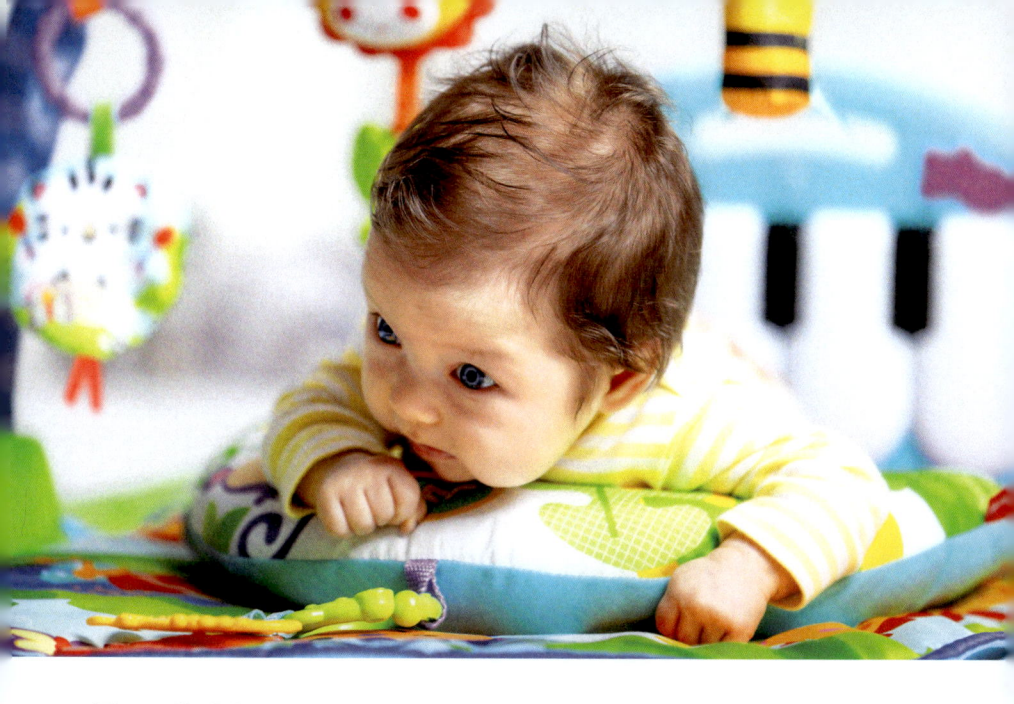

The pull of these muscles on the lower skull, can help to round out the lower part of the back of the head (occipital area).

Lying a baby on his tummy is a great foundation for future milestones and is the step on the path towards rolling, crawling and sitting up. Tummy time also helps develop balance and coordination and is the perfect position later on for baby to explore their environment.

Tummy time should always be supervised. When you start, it may very likely be poorly tolerated as baby may find the position uncomfortable. But as the muscles strengthen, baby will happily spend more time in this position. The trick is to start with just a few minutes at a time and build up slowly. Select a time when baby is content and happy. After a nap and before a feed is ideal when starting out.

Ideas for tummy time

NEWBORN TO THREE MONTHS

- Start tummy time as soon as possible in the first few weeks. The best time is when baby is happy and alert, after a nap perhaps. Avoid tummy time after a feed as baby is likely to spit up.
- To begin with, lay baby belly down across your lap or on your chest.

- Baby may cry at the end of the allotted time as they get tired. Tummy time is hard work for a little baby to begin with.
- As baby gets better at tummy time, you can lie baby on the floor with their arms resting over a rolled-up towel. Get on the floor with baby and have fun.
- Another idea for nearer to three months is to lie baby on an exercise ball and roll the ball gently back and forth. Be sure to hold baby securely and perhaps put a soft blanket under baby.
- Tummy time should last two to three minutes three times a day, building up to this slowly.
- By doing this, your baby will develop better head control and upper body strength.

THREE TO FIVE MONTHS

- By three months your baby will be getting stronger and will be able to lift themselves with their forearms when lying belly down.
- Use toys and mirrors to engage with them during tummy time. This will make it feel more like play time rather than hard work for baby.
- There are plenty of baby gyms that you can buy for this age baby to assist with tummy time. They have raised sides to lean baby over and a selection of toys to entertain baby.
- Ensure you include plenty of face-to-face tummy time and eye contact during this daily routine.
- As baby gets stronger, they will begin to push up onto their extended arms. This prepares them for crawling and sitting.

SIX TO NINE MONTHS

- As baby is now much stronger you can play different games with them as they are better at supporting their head and upper body.

- Play "Airplane" where you lift baby up while supporting their hips and waist.

If Plagiocephaly is present after twelve weeks

If the head flattening persists and is severe enough, the baby may need to see a paediatric physiotherapist for specific exercises and treatment. The physiotherapist will show you how to do the exercises best suited to the type of plagiocephaly your baby has, and you then do the exercises at home.

Sometimes babies can be treated with a helmet (cranial moulding orthosis) to help guide future skull formation. The helmet is non-invasive and works by applying a gentle constant pressure over the areas of your baby's skull which are most prominent while allowing unrestricted growth over the flattened areas. It is a pain-free treatment. The band consists of a soft foam layer inside a thermoplastic shell. This allows for frequent adjustments during growth and gently guides your baby's skull into a more symmetrical shape. The helmet allows your baby to sleep in any position he/she wants by keeping the pressure off the flattened areas.

How paediatric osteopathy can help plagiocephaly and torticollis

Cranial osteopathy may be helpful if plagiocephaly is detected before twelve weeks old. After this time there may be very little benefit unless baby has an unresolved torticollis. In this case, treatment of the neck muscles may help the child.

A cranial osteopath will check the position of the baby's skull alignment with the neck and will evaluate the tension in the neck muscles. The sooner the baby is diagnosed, and preventive measures started, the better the outcome for baby. Cranial osteopathy combined with the above preventive measures is the treatment of choice for babies under twelve weeks old.

Sam's story

Sam is eight weeks old. I had a very long labour with him, and he was finally delivered by forceps as we were both so tired. He's a very happy and contented baby but I had noticed that there was a flat patch at the back of his head. I brought him to see Frank and he explained that this was a condition called plagiocephaly. He checked him over and said that the muscles

on one side of his neck were a little tight and that as a result, Sam was turning his head to one side only. I had not noticed that but once he said it, it looked so obvious.

Frank recommended a special pillow for Sam and gave me tips about how to encourage him to look to the other side. I had tried tummy time with Sam, but he didn't like it and again Frank gave me some ideas to make it a little more comfortable for Sam.

We returned a few weeks later and even Frank was surprised at how improved his head shape was. He had settled into tummy time and was moving his head much better.

Ear infections and glue ear

The ear is made up of three distinct parts: the outer ear, the middle ear (behind the ear drum) and the inner ear (deep within the temporal bone). Ear infections are the most common illness to affect pre-school children with up to 90% of children experiencing one before their third birthday.

When an ear infection occurs, it is the middle ear which is affected. Some children just get the occasional ear infection, others get recurring ear infections and it's generally these children we see at the clinic. They may also go on to develop glue ear as a result of fluid building up in the middle ear.

The middle ear is normally filled with air and is connected to the back of the nasal passages by a small tube called the Eustachian tube. This tube is short and narrow and horizontal in babies and therefore not so effective. As a child grows the tube becomes more oblique and this allows fluid to drain from the middle ear much more effectively. This explains why some parents are often told that their child will "grow out" of ear infections.

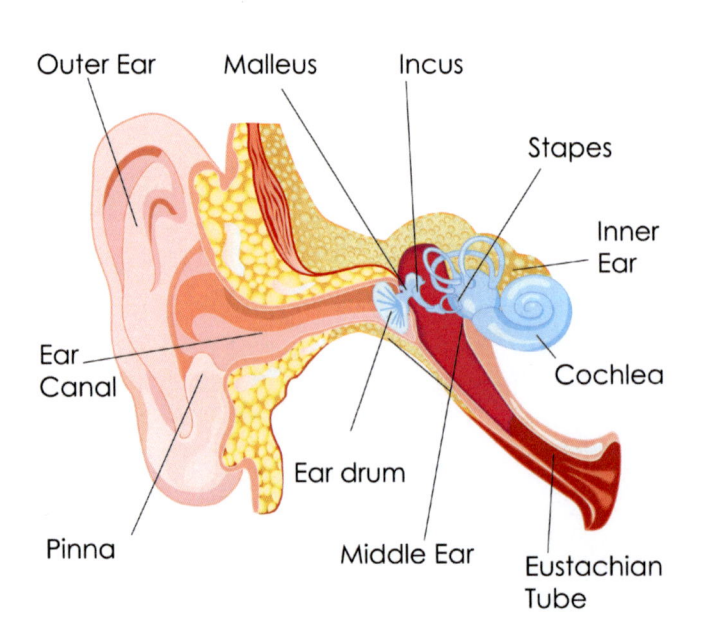

The Eustachian tube allows us to equalise the pressure on either side of the ear drum – like when your ears go pop in a plane. Babies do this by crying, swallowing and yawning. However, when a child is susceptible to coughs, colds and ear infections this tube often becomes inflamed and can be blocked with mucus.

Children are frequently brought to see us because they don't sleep. On closer examination, we sometimes find that the child has had a few ear infections. In many cases like this, the child wakes at night because of the fluid in the middle ear. It may be uncomfortable, and the ears may need to pop. A little drink of water may help when they wake up, but the main aim of treatment is to move the fluid and mucus away from the middle ear, relieving the pressure behind the eardrum.

There are certain conditions that increase the risk of ear infections and glue ear.

- Being under three years of age or being a boy.

- Going to nursery. Children in day-care have more contact with other children and as a result are more likely to catch infections.

- Bottle-fed babies. Breastmilk increases the baby's immune system.

- Being near second-hand smoke. Children with a parent who smokes are 50% more likely to get ear infections and 40% more likely to get glue ear.

- Being in a large family or having a family history of glue ear.

- Using a soother. Children diagnosed with an ear infection have almost double the risk of recurrent infections if they use a soother. Sucking on a soother increases the negative pressure in the Eustachian tube and this draws mucus into the tube.

- Having recurrent coughs and colds and babies who are constantly chesty.

Research done in the Czech Republic and published in the International Journal of Pediatric Otorhinolaryngology in 2015 suggests that there

While soothers can be very useful in babies under six months old, it's advisable to reduce their use after this age.

may be a link between infant reflux and glue ear. In the study, they tested the fluid in the middle ear for the presence of pepsinogen (an enzyme only found in the stomach) during grommet insertion. They discovered that samples from 31.8% of children were positive for pepsinogen.

In babies the Eustachian tube is not fully developed; it's shorter and more horizontal than in adults. As a result, refluxed acidic stomach contents may enter the Eustachian tube and reach the middle ear. This increases the risk of ear infections and glue ear in babies with severe reflux.

Signs and symptoms of an ear infection

Ear infections can be caused by a viral or bacterial infection and very often follow on from a sore throat, cough or cold. Signs and symptoms of an ear infection include high temperature, pain and irritability, nausea and vomiting, difficulty sleeping and the child will often pull at their ears.

In some cases, the ear infection does not clear up completely and this may lead to fluid developing in the middle ear. This in turn will progress on to another ear infection, which exacerbates the problem by increasing the inflammation in the Eustachian tube.

Small children may not be able to tell you they have pain or discomfort and may be seen tugging at their ears. Children with symptoms of an ear infection should always be seen by their doctor.

Types of ear infection

Acute Otitis Media – This is the most common type of ear infection. Fluid builds up behind the eardrum and causes pain. When a very severe infection is present, the eardrum may perforate due to the pressure of the fluid in the middle ear. If this happens, you should see your doctor.

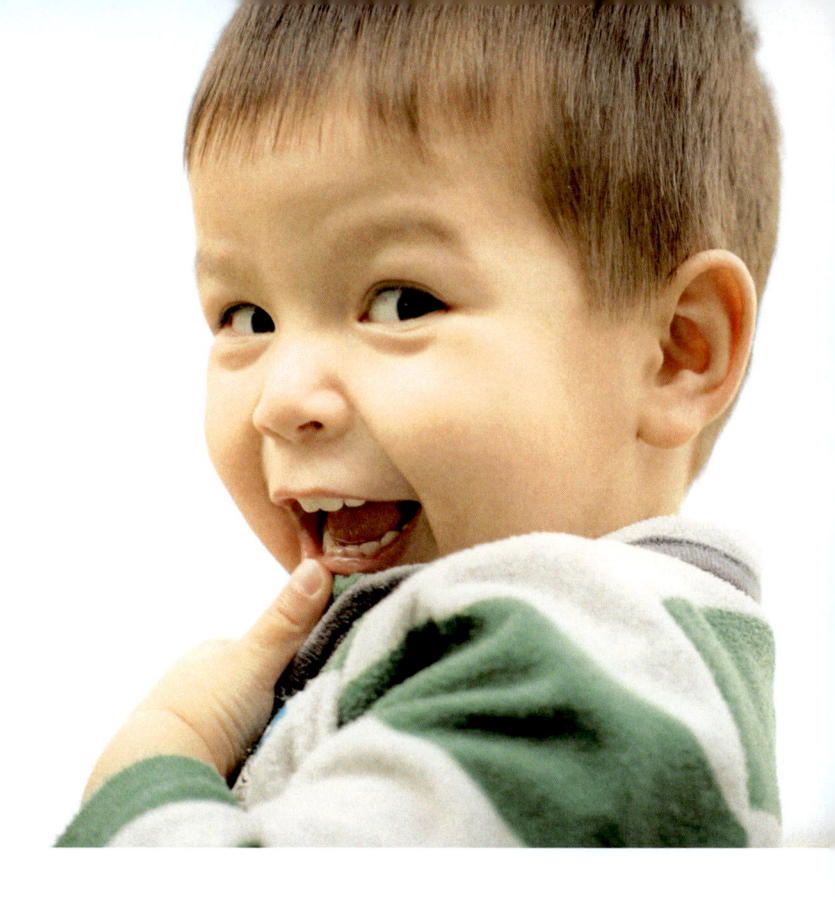

Otitis Media with Effusion – This is more commonly known as glue ear. In this case, fluid remains behind the eardrum after the infection has cleared. This can affect the child's hearing and poses a risk to another infection developing.

Treatment of ear infections

For many infections the main treatment is to manage the symptoms. Give your child an analgesic like paracetamol to relieve the pain and bring down their temperature. Always follow the manufacturer's dosage guidelines and only give the medication when needed.

If the symptoms persist for longer than 48 hours, or if you are concerned about your child, see your doctor. An antibiotic may be needed to treat the infection. You should however always see you doctor if your child's temperature is above 38 degrees Celsius, if they are very distressed or if you have any other concerns.

A cold compress on the affected ear will help reduce the pain.

Encourage your child to drink plenty of fluids, particularly if they have a high temperature.

For children who have a recurring ear infection, it may be worth asking your doctor about antibiotic drops instead of oral antibiotics.

Glue ear

Glue ear is essentially fluid behind the eardrum. This fluid builds up as a result of recurring ear infections. The tube that should drain the fluid from the middle ear, the Eustachian tube, can become inflamed and blocked. Over time, this fluid may become thick (hence the name – glue) and cause discomfort, and can also affect the child's hearing. Imagine hearing everything with water in your ears! That is what it sounds like for a child with glue ear.

While ear infections are easy to diagnose, glue ear can be more difficult. Sound waves travel through the ear by vibrating the eardrum and then these vibrations are transferred to three tiny bones in the middle ear and then to the inner ear where the vibrations are interpreted as sound. If the middle ear contains fluid rather than air, the movement of the sound waves through this area to the inner ear is affected.

Very often, if glue ear is a persistent problem, the child's speech and hearing may be affected and this in turn can lead to behavioural issues as they become frustrated. Audiology tests are important as they will both confirm the presence of fluid behind the ear drum and test the child's hearing.

Audiology testing will include a tympanometry test, which measures how well the eardrum can move. If there is fluid in the middle ear the eardrum will not work properly. A hearing test will also be done to check if the glue ear is affecting your child's hearing and if so, by how much.

Look out for the following if you think your child may have glue ear:

- No reply when called
- TV turned up loud
- Complains of ear pain or discomfort
- Speech is delayed
- Lack of concentration
- Balance issues or clumsiness
- In school going children they may begin to fall behind at school

Paediatric osteopathy can help drain this fluid from the ears. It is a wonderful first option treatment as it is so gentle. As winter approaches, we always begin to see more children with ear infections as a result of the usual coughs and colds picked up at that time of year. Many parents also bring their children back for check-ups to keep them healthy over the winter.

Another helpful idea is an *Otovent* auto-inflation device. This is suitable for children who are old enough to blow their nose. The aim of the device is to inflate the balloon with the nose. The balloons are included in the kit and are specially pressurised. This action helps to open the Eustachian tubes allowing the fluid associated with glue ear to safely drain away.

Sometimes grommets may need to be inserted by an ENT doctor to assist the drainage. This is a very minor surgical procedure done under a general anaesthetic where a small incision is made in the ear drum and little plastic tubes are inserted to allow fluid to drain. Children who have grommets inserted should avoid getting water in their ears. Precautions should be taken when swimming and at bath-time.

A great product for swimming is the *Ear Band-It Ultra* headband which was invented by an Ear Nose and Throat (ENT) physician. This headband will hold earplugs in place while the child is swimming.

Occasionally the grommets can fall out. If this happens, the eardrum heals naturally itself.

How paediatric osteopathy can help ear infections and glue ear

As a paediatric osteopath, I treat children with recurrent ear infections and glue ear frequently. Firstly, I examine the available movement in their temporal bones; these are the bones at the side of the skull in which the ear is located. I observe the position of the temporal bones compared to each other and compared to the occipital bone at the back of the skull.

Flat headedness in babies may affect the movement of the ear bones and the adjacent bones of the skull. Babies who have had a forceps delivery are more likely to have increased tension in the temporal bones due to the pressure applied during delivery.

By reducing the tension in the temporal bones, the function of the Eustachian tube is improved and this in turn helps fluid to drain from the middle ear. I also examine upper rib cage movement and the tension in the muscles that connect the ribs to the ear bone surfaces, as many ear infections originate in the upper respiratory tract as a result of coughs and colds.

Successful treatment must also include the doctor, as ear infections may continue to occur occasionally. The fluid in the middle ear is thick and mucousy and can take time to drain. However, over time, the ear infections become less frequent and the glue ear begins to resolve.

Sadie's story

Sadie was a great baby. She had a little reflux but that seemed to settle down after a few months. A week after her first birthday she got an ear infection and needed antibiotics. She recovered quickly but after three weeks she got another one. This was the start of her getting ear infections every six weeks or so. Her sleep got worse too and she had been a great sleeper.

After her sixth antibiotic I brought her to see Frank. He told me that she had some fluid behind her eardrum and that this was very likely causing the repeated infections. He treated her three times over a six week period and after the second treatment, she started sleeping through the night again. She was so much happier and thankfully has not had another ear infection since.

Mark's story

Mum brought Mark to see me when he was three years old. She said that Mark had got his first ear infection at eighteen months old and to date, was just finishing his ninth antibiotic. She was down to visit the doctorGP service every three to four weeks.

I asked Mum to tell me Mark's story. He had reflux from six weeks to six months but when he went on solids it eased. He was a very poor sleeper and only started sleeping through the night at two years. He had persistent congestion, waxy ears, runny nose and a night-time cough. He had a tough teething process, lots of dribbling, chewing, red cheeks and wakeful nights and would fall a lot when learning to walk. He had up to ten to twelve ear infections at this stage, some of them viral, others bacterial with a discharge from his ear.

The key here was the recurrent nature of the ear infections. I asked Mum about any family history of ear infections. Dad had grommets as a child and a first cousin also had to have grommets inserted. In my experience there is often a previous family history in children with recurring ear infections and glue ear. It's worth asking the question at case history.

I treated Mark at the clinic over a period of six weeks, three treatments in total. I focused treatment on the respiratory system, activation of ribcage, lengthening of musculature of the neck, deepening the breathing and improve the ear surface motion to help Eustachian tube drainage.

I advised Mum to undertake a decongestion home plan. This involved giving Mark probiotics to strengthen his immune

system response, using a Salin salt pump at night to decongest and dry up mucous, and decreasing diary intake and substitute with other fortified diary sources. I suggested a GP visit to the doctor to check ear integrity.

I reviewed Mark after six weeks. He was ear infection-free, less congested and healthy. If the plan hadn't worked and Mark's response was poor, I would have asked his Mum to contact his doctorGP to get a referral to an Ear Nose and NThroat consultant because in my opinion a family history of ear infections can be significant as some children may inherit smaller Eustachian tubes than others.

Behaviour, anxiety and concentration

Getting distracted is normal for young children and most children have times when they are restless and forgetful. Busy days, sleepless nights and ill health all take their toll on small children. In general, the most common causes for lack of concentration among children include tiredness and late nights, poor diet and lack of parental interest.

When necessary however, most children will be able to concentrate on a task and complete it, be that task tidying their room, reading a book or doing their homework. Being able to concentrate means that children can keep their minds focused on a task for a reasonable period of time, the length of time depending on the age of the child.

If your child is fidgety and unable to sit and concentrate for long, and you have out ruled the obvious causes of distraction, it may be due to physical discomfort and tension that they do not have the words to explain. As some children retain the stresses and strains of birth, gentle treatment from a trained cranial osteopath can be beneficial to help release these pressures, enabling your child to fully engage with life again. A child who is physically uncomfortable may not complain of aches and pains. The stresses have probably been present since birth and have become "normal" for that child.

They may however be affected at a subtle level and display any or all the following characteristics:

Illnesses: The child often has a lower immune system and gets frequent infections.

Learning can be detrimentally affected by both a child feeling unwell and increased time lost from school.

Retained birth moulding in the head restricts the development of the nasal sinuses and the ears. Such children are vulnerable to chronic ear infections and glue ear, with associated loss of hearing that can delay speech development and interfere with classroom learning.

They are often habitual mouth breathers.

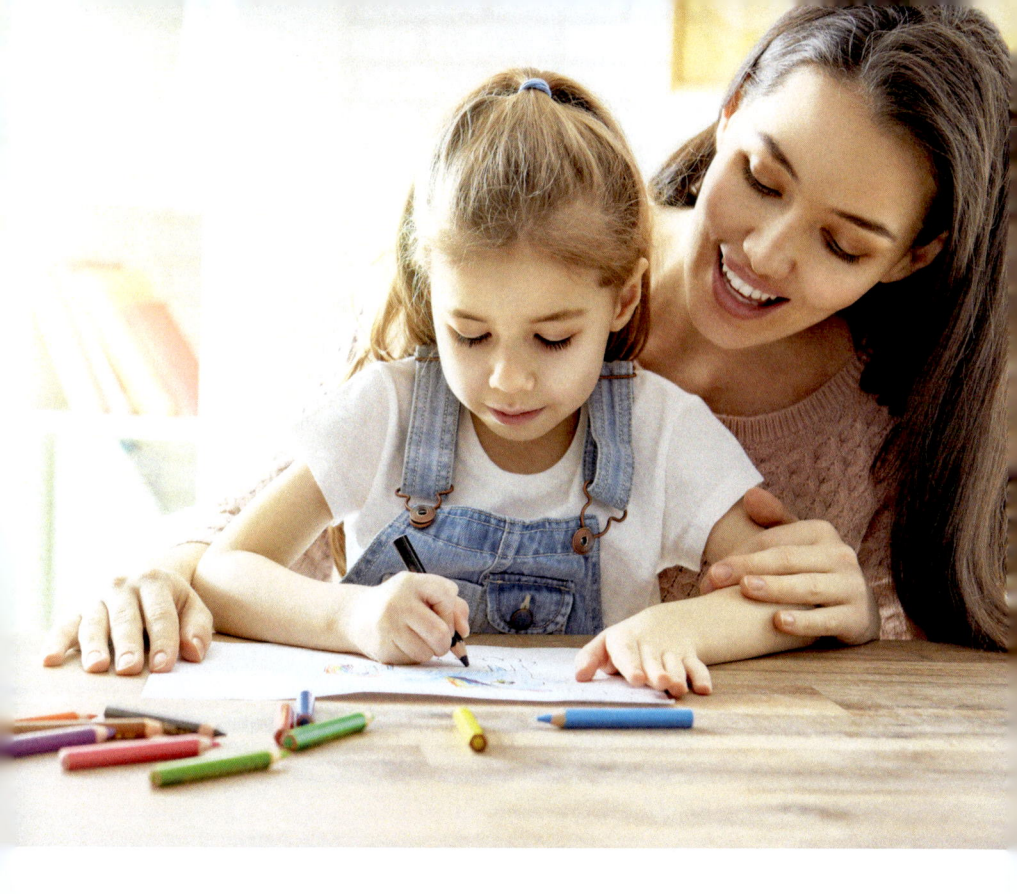

Physical signs: There may be asymmetries in the child's posture, such as holding the head on one side, or one shoulder being higher than the other.

It may be easier for the child to turn to one side than the other. This has implications on the best seating position within the classroom, to allow for activities such as watching the teacher, copying from the blackboard etc.

Physical discomforts: The child may complain of headaches, growing pains, stomach aches or other physical aches and pains.

Sensory issues: Sensory processing refers to how the brain receives messages from the senses, and then provides a response appropriate to the situation. Children with sensory processing difficulties are often restless and fidgety.

Signs to look out for include:

- On the go/unable to sit still
- Twirls/spins excessively
- Over responsive to touch/sound/light/smells
- Takes excessive risks during play
- Doesn't like standing near others, e.g. in a line
- Difficulty winding down for bed
- Picky eater – doesn't like food textures to mix or can only tolerate a particular type of food, crunchy or smooth.

Tips to improve your child's concentration

Promote a healthy diet: children can sometimes have an unbalanced diet with a preponderance of processed foods, saturated fats and sugary foods. Studies have shown that a diet rich in whole grains, fruits and veggies will help your child's brain functions. Also, studies have shown that children should avoid foods that have food colouring in them, as they may increase hyperactivity, something most parents will have proof of themselves.

Set routines: children need to have a routine (time for meals, school, homework), a ritual of things to do. Figure out a regular routine that will suit you and your child. Displaying the daily routine on a chart or white board at home can be helpful for more visual children or those who like to know what's happening next.

Limit the use of television and electronics: too much TV and computer games can prevent children from doing activities like, reading, doing homework, playing outside and interacting with friends and with family. At a time when we are surrounded by electronic devices, this can be a little difficult to achieve. Be consistent and persistent and you will be successful.

Exercise more often: both mental and physical exercise are very important to help your child concentrate better. For mental exercises, try playing board games that stimulate your child to think strategically and focus, guessing games, or even allowing them to help you cook by reading or following recipes. For physical exercise, it has been scientifically proven that children who do at least 30 minutes of exercise per day are more likely to do well in school, focus better and generally be more positive.

Support your child: if at all possible, be there to support your child when they come home from school with homework. Sit down and help them as they do the task and give them encouragement and support.

Be honest and open with your child: your children pick up on everything whether you believe they do or not. If something is going on within the family, talk to your child about his or her feelings. Try to explain in simple terms what is happening without adding to their worry.

How paediatric osteopathy can help improve behaviour and concentration

When working with children who have focus & concentration issues, it is noticeable that they often have difficulty in being still and at ease. When treatment begins you notice that the child is moving a lot and their breathing is changing.

The treatment orientates the child to begin to breathe more deeply by releasing tension in the muscular system through the ribcage and neck area and then, allows the breathing diaphragm space to lengthen. Finally, the cranium (skull) is orientated to a neutral position by gently balancing the muscular tension of the upper neck muscles. This allows the child to breathe deeply and relax the nervous system response. It has a calming effect for the child.

Samuel's story

Sam was eleven days overdue and was born by vacuum and forceps weighing in at 9lb and 8oz. For the first few days he was a little stunned but the paediatrician said it was the shock of the birth.

Sam was always a lively little boy and got himself into the usual "boy" things. He reached all his normal milestones and was a happy little toddler. When he began pre-school, he was a nervous little child and knew how to play up to "mother" but there was always some little thing with Sam that needed extra attention.

He started primary school at four years and nine months and the first year went well. It was in senior infants that his teacher noticed something wasn't quite right with Sam. We organised the normal assessments and apart from sensory issues, Sam seemed to pass all the tests. Reading and writing and general little things were a problem for Sam. He couldn't grasp these subjects, but his mind could retain facts about History and Geography that would surprise you.

After attending another set of assessments his clinical psychologist still couldn't find a "label" or "diagnosis" for Sam as he was a great child on a one-to-one basis. But put him into a classroom situation and he seemed to drift off and lose concentration and basically fall behind.

I brought Sam to see Frank that spring. His head was all tight on the right side and his breathing was very erratic and fast for his age. I have to say from day one Sam seemed to be improving before my very eyes. I said nothing to his teacher until our four treatments were over, just to see if he would notice a difference. I had a brief chat with him, and his first words were "Sam is really flying at the moment. What's the story?" The words I was waiting for!

Sam had a break then until July where we re-checked how things were going and Frank said what he had done stayed in place. Sam is now back at school after the summer break and so far, so good. His concentration is good, his form is great and he seems so well able to deal with things.

Katie's story

Mum brought Katie to see me when she was six years old. Mum said that Katie was the youngest of three children. She had an older brother nine years old and sister seven years old. Mum said Katie had a difficult birth after a very short labour of four hours. Baby got distressed, had heart rate fluctuation, had the cord around her neck and needed a little oxygen after delivery. She was fine afterwards and fed very well from the beginning.

Mum said Katie had developed a poor sleeping pattern from about eight months on, needing someone to be with her until she went to sleep and still required Mum or Dad to settle her to sleep at night. She would still come into her parent's bed to sleep at least once a week.

Katie had the typical temper tantrums from two to three years, however Mum said that it took longer to calm her down afterwards. Mum said that Katie was restless, wanting to be on the go all the time, and would lose her cool with her siblings very quickly.

When school began, Katie initially found the transition difficult, lots of crying going to school in the morning, and even refusing to go in some days. Her teacher said that once she was in school, Katie was very sociable, with lots of friends. She was good academically but found sitting still to complete a task difficult at times.

Mum said that Katie took her time to join in new activities when they went on social events and would watch for a while close to Mum before joining in.

I treated Katie for several weeks based on what Mum had told me. In my experience, when treating kids that present like Katie, it is important to note that behaviour is linked to concentration and anxiety. The key to treatment is to observe the child's actions in treatment. My attention is based on influencing the respiratory system, lengthening the breathing and easing tension in the anatomy of this system,

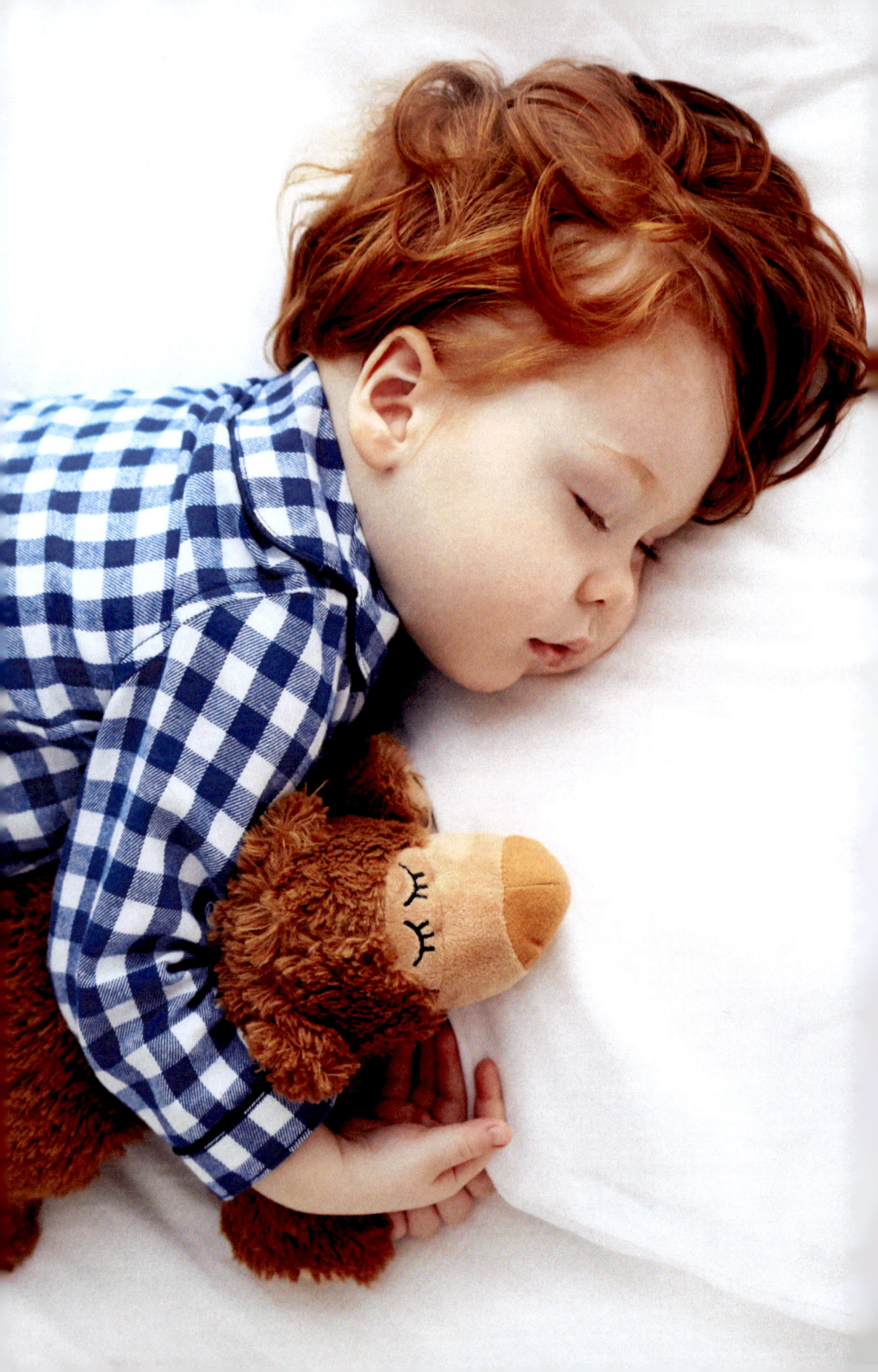

Night terrors

Children often wake up upset after having a bad dream or nightmare. In general, they can be settled and soothed and will go off back to sleep again. With night terrors it's very different. Night terror is a very big term for what is essentially a type of bad dream. The child will cry out and will be visibly distressed but is still sound asleep. They may shout out for you but can't sense your presence or be comforted by you, making it difficult to sooth and reassure your child. They will return to sleep after a period of between 1–30 minutes but will not usually remember the details in the morning (although you will!)

While nightmares occur from dream sleep (rapid eye-movement or REM sleep), night terrors occur from a deep non-dream sleep. A child may be able to recall a nightmare if they wake up, but a child experiencing a night terror is not fully awake and will not remember the event.

Night terrors are common in children between the ages of three to eight years old. The episode usually happens early in the night and they are more common in children with a family history of night terrors or sleepwalking.

Night terrors in a child are probably more distressing for the parents than they are for the child. They can occur after a traumatic event like a fall or a hospital admission, because of a change of schedule, a new baby in the house or stress or anxiety about something in your child's life, or if a child is overtired and falls into a very deep sleep very quickly.

Our experience of a night terror was when our oldest son was about four years old. He was sick and had a fever. While it was very distressing, both for him and for us, thankfully it never happened again. We understand how parents can feel helpless when it comes to recurring night terrors. And we love to see the change that children and parents experience after paediatric osteopathy treatment.

> *Night terrors usually happen early in the night and can be more distressing for the parents than they are for the child.*

	NIGHT TERROR	NIGHTMARE
Time of night	Early, usually within four hours of going to sleep	Later in the night
How child acts	Child can be confused, agitated and disorientated	Frightened and upse
Child's response to parents	Is not aware of parent's presence and therefore cannot be comforted by them	Is awake so can be comforted
Memory of event	Usually none	Can remember the dream
Return to sleep	Usually quick, unless the child has been woken up	Often slow as the child may be afraid
Sleep Stage	Deep non-REM sleep	Light REM sleep

Symptoms of a night terror

- Wakes suddenly from a deep sleep and gets very agitated
- Child may look like they are awake with their eyes open
- Crying and upset
- May get out of bed and run around
- Usually happens early in the night
- Increased heart rate
- Increased breathing rate
- Sweating

What can cause a night terror?

In many cases there's often a reason why night terrors occur. As adults, we can take everyday things that happen to us in our stride. A child can often have a very different reaction. We have seen children who have had a minor injury that required a hospital visit, to later develop night terrors. Or a new baby and a change in routine at home can be the cause.

Of course, not every child will react this way to normal everyday events. And sometimes, there's not an obvious reason. As children get older and can rationalise their world better, the likelihood of night terrors will decrease.

What to do

- Do not try to wake your child as they will be very confused and disorientated if they do wake up.
- Remain calm and wait for the night terror to burn itself out. This can take anything up to 30 minutes.
- Keep your child safe during this time as they may be thrashing about.
- Once over, guide your child back into bed and they will continue their nights' sleep.

Night terrors will settle in time with reassurance but because they can be so distressing, many parents will look for a solution. Cranial osteopathy is a very gentle treatment that works on the child's nervous system and breathing diaphragm and is a very effective way to treat night terrors successfully.

How paediatric osteopathy can help night terrors

When treating a child that presents with a night terror, it is important to find out if there was a recent stressful event. The key to treatment is to recognise the restriction in movement of the ribcage, particularly the activation of both the pump handle and bucket handle action. Breathing is a coordination of both those actions. When a child wakes with a night terror they are often agitated, and their breathing pattern is more rapid.

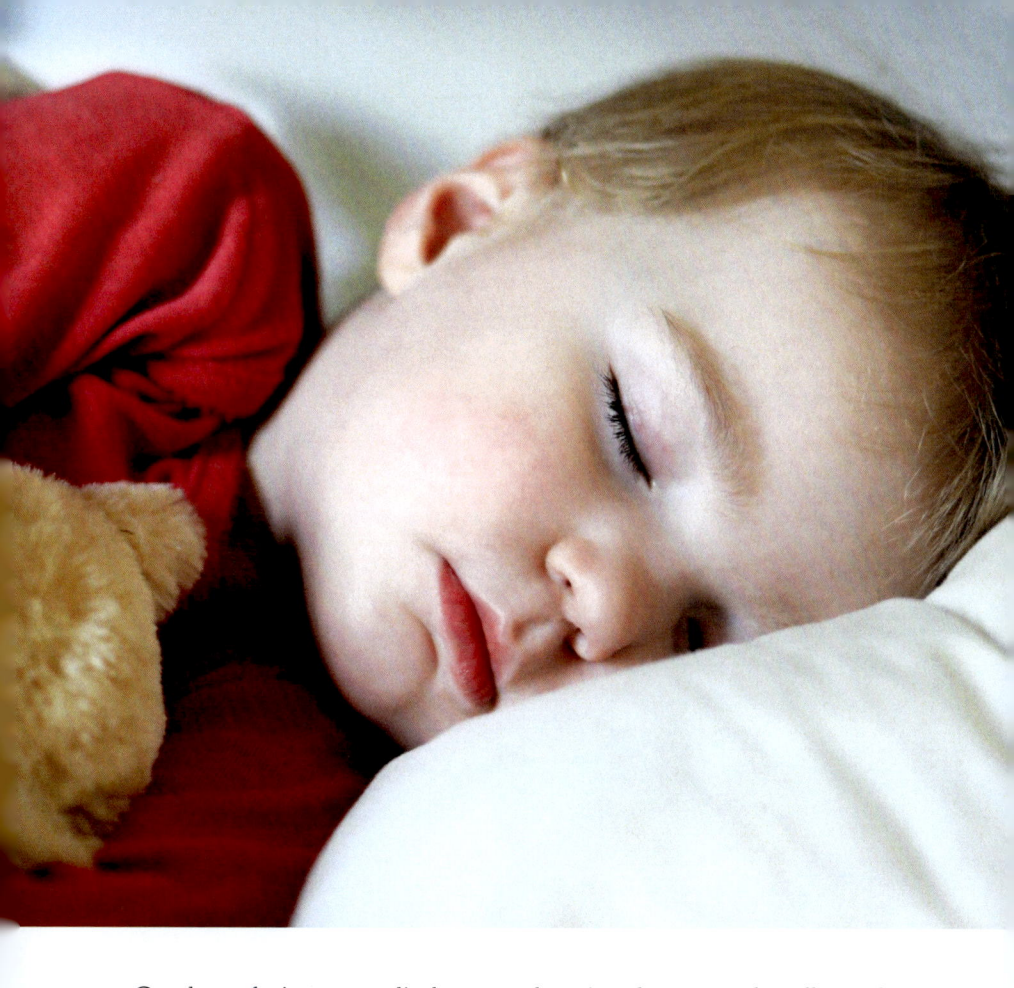

Gentle techniques applied to synchronise the pump handle and bucket handle action of the ribcage allows a lengthening of the breathing diaphragm and a deepening of the breath. Pump handle action occurs in the upper ribcage and is an upward movement of the ribs. Bucket handle motion occurs in the lower ribcage and is rib movements to the sides. These are the movements that happen when a child breaths in. This, in my view, rebalances the nervous system response. The child then has an improved sleeping pattern, which eliminates night terrors. The breath is the key.

Katie' story

Katie had a fall off her bike a few months ago and needed a few stitches in a head wound. She was kept in hospital overnight just as a precaution. After a week or so she was back to her best. However, about three weeks after her fall she started waking in the night, shouting out, terrified! She would look around the room and not even see us. After about ten minutes she would calm down and fall back to sleep. The funny thing was that she couldn't remember anything about it the next day!

I think I found it more upsetting than she did to be honest. This would happen about three to four times a week and after two weeks I decided to bring her to Frank.

She loved the treatment. After just one treatment the frequency of the night terrors decreased and after the second treatment, she was a different child.

Down's Syndrome

This chapter focuses on the benefits of osteopathic treatment for children with Down's Syndrome (DS). Frank has a special interest in working with DS children. Thirty years ago, he qualified as a nurse for people with intellectual disabilities. He worked in People with Learning Disability (PLD) services and would have assisted children with DS as part of his day-to-day job. He had always hoped to help children with disabilities in his work as an osteopath. His studies of the anatomy of children with DS has focused his attention on a few specific key areas to treat, as the physical features of a DS child can affect their ability to breathe well.

Why a DS child is more susceptible to chest and ear infections

The skull of a child with DS has reduced growth. The main affected areas are in the ethmoid bone (a bone that sits at the top of the nasal passages behind the bridge of the nose), the nasal bones, the maxilla (the bone the top teeth are located in) and the mandible (jaw). This reduced growth gives the child the characteristic facial features of Down's Syndrome. In the DS child's skull there is also an absence in the development of the sphenoid (deep behind the nasal passages) and frontal (forehead) sinuses. The absence of frontal sinuses has a considerable influence on the characteristic shaping of the frontal bones and forehead.

The anatomical ear structure of children with DS has characteristics that may predispose them to hearing deficits. Some hearing issues may be congenital (present at birth) as a result of an inner ear condition. Others can be due to the size of the cochlea (inner ear) and the middle ear structures. This can lead to glue ear and hearing impairment that requires support.

The child with DS can also have musculo-skeletal issues such as hypotonia (low muscle tone). As a result of having respiratory muscles with hypotonia, the clearance of mucous from the respiratory system can be inefficient during an infection. Coughing up mucous can be difficult and this can prolong the recovery.

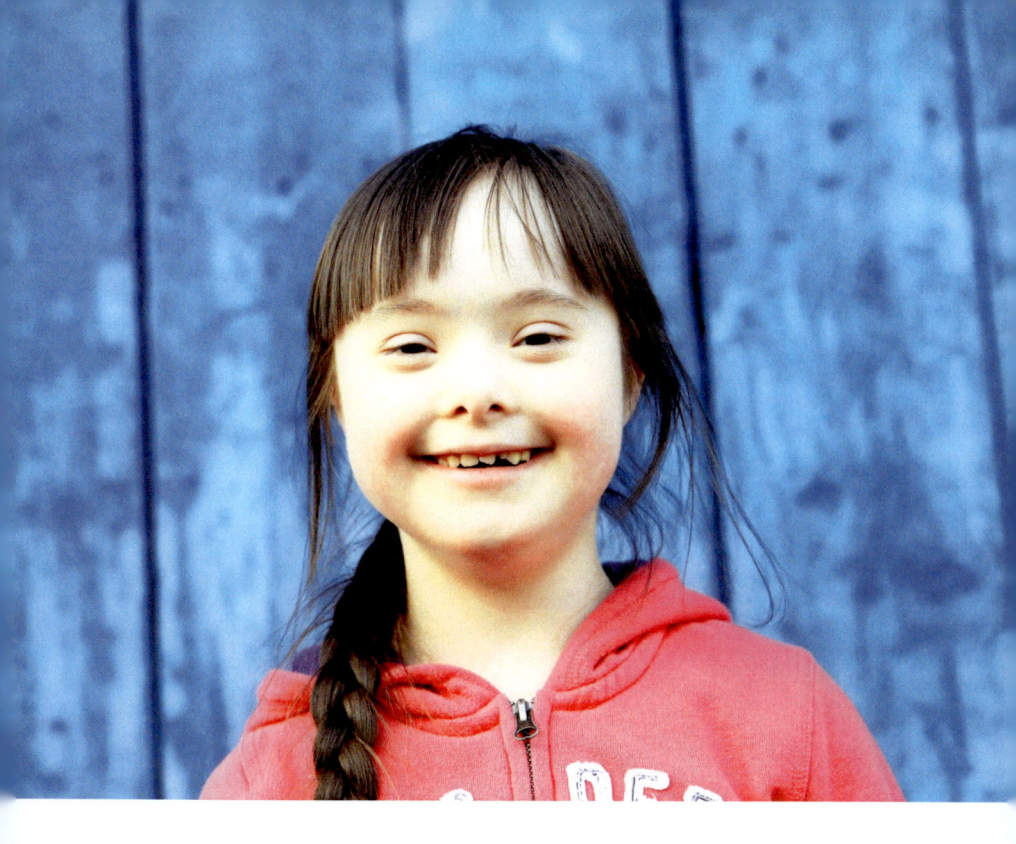

How infection occurs

When I am treating children with DS, I focus on the features above and how they influence the function of the respiratory system. Other factors I take into consideration are airway problems and tongue protrusion with associated oxygen reduction due to mouth breathing.

The consequence of poor sinus development is reduced drainage of mucous from the sinuses, which then pools, thickens and can become a hotbed for infection. The nasal lining becomes inflamed with a copious infected discharge, and the adenoids and tonsils enlarge. Frequently antibiotics are prescribed. They can reduce the infection and discharge but do nothing for the pooling of mucous within the sinuses.

In the DS child, their narrow nasal passages are further narrowed or even blocked by the discharge, forcing the child to breathe through their mouth which is already narrowed by a steeple palate.

Nasal discharge may also track into the middle ear, compromising the draining of mucous through the eustachian tube. This causes a build-up of fluid in the ears (glue ear) affecting hearing. This middle ear mucous may eventually drain on to the tonsils and track down to the bronchial tubes and lead to chest infections. Poor muscle tone in the ribcage may slow down clearance of mucous in the child with DS as their ability to cough up mucous is reduced.This explains why DS children are more susceptible to recurrent infection, requiring repeated antibiotics and often very regular visits to their doctor or hospital admissions.

Treatment

We believe the main principle of treatment is to improve breathing, by improving the drainage of mucous through the sinuses, so that the child can breathe more through their nose. This improves oxygen levels and the tongue will not protrude as much, which in turn reduces fatigue associated with mouth breathing.

Drainage of the middle ear is enhanced as the mucous has now got an exit. The ribcage can then expand due to improved oxygen levels which allows mucous clearance, from the bronchial tubes. The outcome of these improvements should be a decreased number of infections.

Peter's story

Peter, a ten-month-old child with Down's Syndrome, attended the clinic with his Mum. He was born at 38 weeks, naturally. He was checked by the doctors in the hospital and didn't have any heart defects and his respiratory system was healthy.

Mum stated that Peter was formula fed and did very well. He was weaned onto solids at six months and was thriving. He was a good sleeper for the first eight months, but this changed when he got a chest infection. Mum said that after this he appeared constantly congested, with a blocked nose and chesty cough. It was worse at night and was waking him up. He was also pulling at his ears on a regular basis. He was mouth breathing more often and getting tired more easily.

Peter had an audiology test done in the hospital which found fluid in both ears. He was for review at the audiology department again in three months.

The key to treatment here, was to improve breathing through the nasal passageways, reduce mouth breathing, improve ribcage range of movement to clear mucous and to ease the tension in the muscles supporting the base of the skull (cranium) to enhance drainage of mucous through the Eustachian tubes of the ears. These gentle techniques were used for three treatments in a five week period. I also advised Mum to use a salt humidifier in Peter's room to assist mucous drainage.

In the five week period during treatment Peter didn't have any further infection. On return to the clinic Mum said that his mucous levels initially increased for three to four days and then started to subside. His chesty cough had eased, and *he was sleeping better. Mum said she noticed that he was more energetic.*

Two months later Mum called the clinic to say that the audiology tests had been repeated and that they had showed no fluid in his left ear and reduced levels in his right ear. He was infection free in the past two months. My conclusion with this case is that understanding the limitations of the facial bones, treating the total respiratory system musculo-skeletally, and creating mucous draining by enhancing breathing function gives the best outcome for the DS child.

Constipation

Constipation is the passing of hard stools, with difficulty, less often. While every child is different and what's normal can vary, the sooner constipation is recognised and treated the better. Constipation is a very common issue in children, with up to 10% of children experiencing constipation at some stage. It can occur at any age and for a variety of reasons.

A baby's bowel motions may be influenced by several factors. Some babies have a bowel motion initially after every feed, others once a day. Others may take even longer to have a motion. It is dependent on your baby's normal pattern and on what he eats and drinks daily. Other influencing factors are how active your baby is and how quickly their food is digested.

Bowel motions can vary a lot between formula and breastfed babies. Breastfed babies can have one motion a week and that can be a normal pattern for them so long as they are well and gaining weight. Generally, if a baby is taking formula and solids each day, they will have a motion each day. The most important factor to look out for is a change in the normal pattern of your baby. If he hasn't had a motion for three to four days, is uncomfortable trying to do a poo, and if the motion is dry, hard and difficult to pass, then he may be constipated.

We see babies very often with constipation, but it is usually as a result of a feeding issue and once that is resolved, the constipation resolves too. Some examples of the type of feeding issues we see include:

1. Babies who are formula fed and find it difficult to break down the milk proteins (casein) in the formula. These babies require assistance from a health professional to advise them on a formula change where the protein is more digestible.

2. When solid foods are introduced baby can become slightly constipated as the solids increase. Several of the cereal food groups commonly used during weaning are lower in fibre which can contribute to constipation.

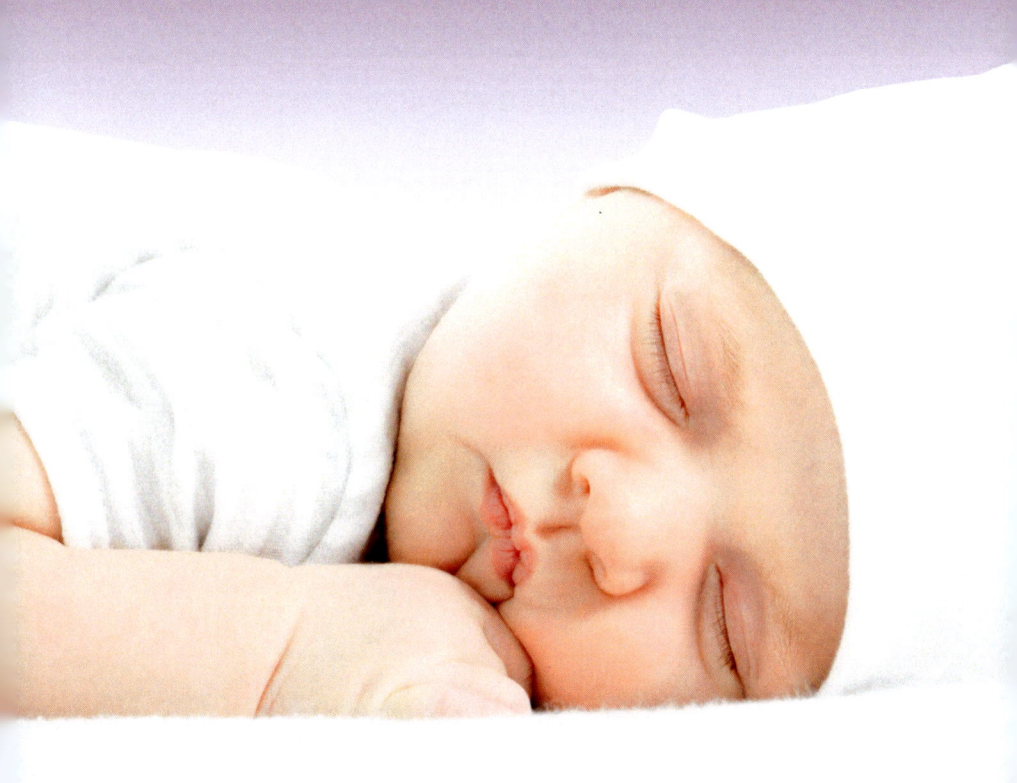

3. When a breast-fed baby is introduced to solids, they can get constipated due to reduction of liquids leading to dehydration.

Top tips for baby

If a baby becomes dehydrated, his digestive system will re-absorb fluid from whatever he eats and drinks. This leads to hard, dry stools that are difficult to pass. If you think your baby is dehydrated or constipated, you can increase their water intake. If you are breast or bottle feeding, you can offer your baby a small drink of cool boiled water after their feed but no more than 2ozs/60mls in 24 hours for babies up to six months old.

If your baby is over six months old, you can offer them fruit juice. Prune, pear or apple are great for getting things going but no more than one teaspoon per 4ozs of cool boiled water.

Baby massage is a wonderful way to connect with your baby and to offer a little help if they are constipated. It's worth doing a class to get the techniques correct and of course, it's also a social morning for mums.

Giving baby a little exercise is helpful if they become constipated. Lie them on their back and pump their legs as if they were pedalling a bike.

Once baby is weaned, offer them a good variety of foods to include a selection of fruit and vegetables. Offering your baby different vegetables every day will increase the likelihood of them liking them as they get older, and of course they are packed with fibre, so it's a win-win! As baby gets older, choose a ripe piece of fruit rather than a puree pouch, as the whole fruit will contain more nutrients and fibre and less free sugar. Ripe fruit makes excellent finger food.

Causes of constipation in older children

Firstly, lets explain how things work. When a child eats a meal, a signal is sent from the stomach to the colon to prepare it for a bowel motion. It can take up to one hour for a child to feel the full effect of this. After the food is eaten, it leaves the stomach and travels through the digestive system where it sits in the lower gut while waiting for a bowel motion to happen. The rectum sends a signal to the brain that it is time for a bowel motion but while the child goes to a bathroom, an involuntary muscle holds things in. Only when the child is sitting on the toilet will this muscle relax allowing the child to open their bowels. It sounds simple, but it's a complex sequence of events requiring muscles to co-ordinate and the right signals to be sent and received. This starts to happen at age three to four years.

Diet – Eating foods that are high in fat and low in fibre may cause constipation. Fast food and sugary drinks are the worst culprits here. A high intake of milk where the child is not eating enough solids can also cause constipation due to a lack of fibre. Drinking water is essential for growing children and should therefore be encouraged.

Lack of exercise – Exercise is a great way to move the digested food through the gut. A child who spends most of their time sedentary will be at a higher risk of developing constipation.

Time – Busy children don't pay attention to the signs their bodies give them about needing to poo. They forget to go as they are too busy playing. This can also be an issue for children starting school where they may need to ask to use the bathroom. School days are busy and full of fun with lunch breaks packed with eating and play.

It's good to identify a "go" time for your child. Pick a time when you can support them in the early stages, and you are not too rushed with other children/tasks. This helps a child to recognise their body cues and reinforces good toileting habits.

Emotional issues – Toilet training can be a difficult time for children. Accidents will happen from time to time. How you react to these accidents will be important in determining your child's reaction to potty training. Keep calm and reassure them. This will let them know that they have not done anything wrong and therefore the occasional accident will not affect their confidence.

Some children are a little more sensitive about using the bathroom than others. They may require more privacy and may prefer to wait till they get home from crèche or school. By then, the urge may have passed. Toddlers can also intentionally hold back a poo when in a power struggle with Mum or Dad. Older children who are stressed may also develop constipation.

Other physical problems – Some underlying issues, including problems with the lower bowel, rectum or anus, can cause constipation. Children who have hypothyroidism, cerebral palsy or who are on certain medications such as iron can get constipation. However, up to 90% of cases of constipation are functional, with no medical cause.

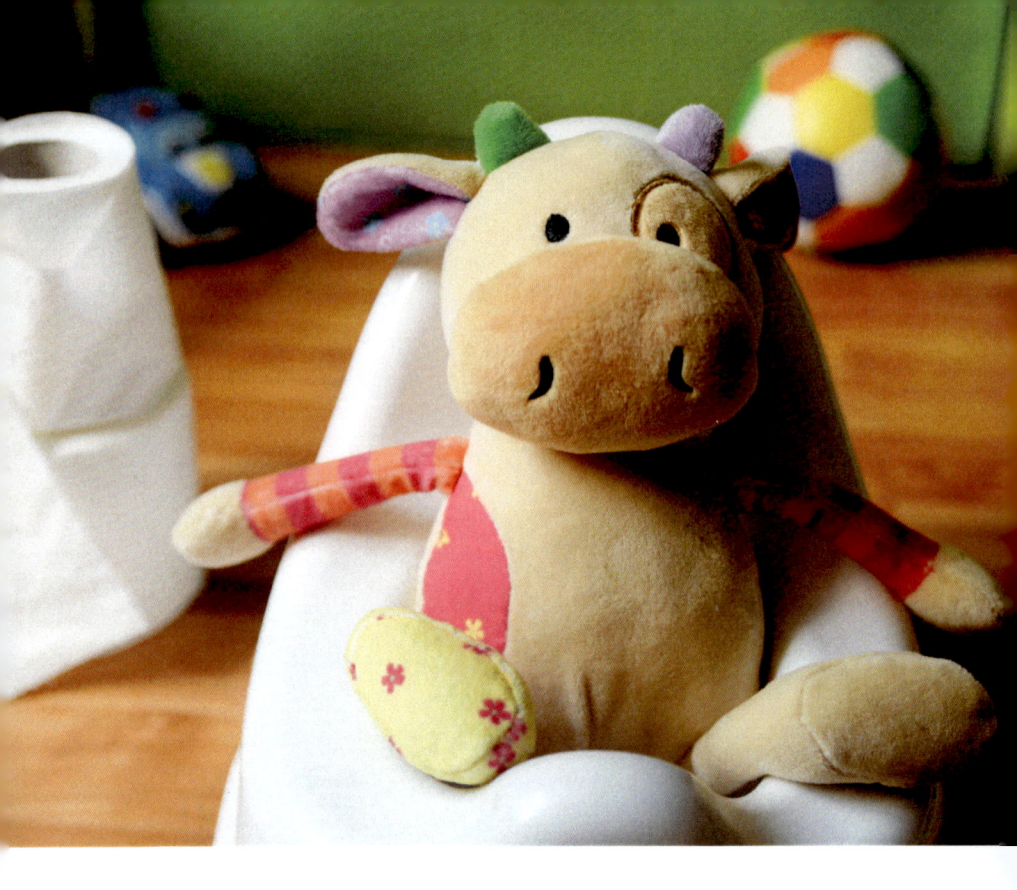

Symptoms of constipation

- Reduction in the frequency of bowel movements
- Straining when passing a stool
- Passing hard stools
- Pain when passing a stool
- Complaining of tummy pain
- Not feeling hungry
- Feeling sick
- Restlessness
- Impaction

In cases of severe constipation, a child may suffer from impaction. This is where a large hard stool is stuck in the lower rectum. This can cause the child to soil themselves with soft faeces that pushes past the impacted stool and leaks out. Parents sometimes mistake this for diarrhoea. Although it may seem like diarrhoea, the child is constipated and needs to be treated for this.

Laxatives

This is the usual treatment for constipation. Laxatives are prescribed by your doctor as a sachet of powder that is mixed with a drink. *Movicol* is the drug of choice for most children. Dosage depends on the age of the child and the severity of the constipation. Treatment can continue for quite a while, depending on each child. Some children will continue to experience abdominal pain when on Movicol and waiting for the bowel to clear. Once this happens, the dosage may be adjusted down by your doctor. The child should continue using Movicol for a period of time to allow the muscles and the nerves of the lower bowel to recover and to promote regular bowel motions and good toileting habits. Movicol should not be stopped suddenly but should be reduced gradually while monitoring the bowel motions.

Top tips for the older child

Make sure your child is well hydrated. Offer them plenty of drinks, mainly water. Monitor their water intake, as most parents would be surprised how little a constipated child drinks every day. Avoid sugary drinks. Milk can contribute to constipation so keep their intake balanced.

A child's diet is important for treating and preventing constipation. Plenty of fruit and vegetables every day. Offer different types and tastes and encourage them to get involved in the preparation.

Exercise is essential for every child but especially for a child prone to constipation as it helps to stimulate normal bowel movement.

Have a routine for bowel habits. After breakfast is a good time but be sure to allow plenty of time so that your child is not rushed, and you have time to sit with them if needed. Allow them to sit on the toilet for five minutes. Explain about what the sensation of needing to do a poo feels like and reassure them that it's ok. Make sure your child can rest their feet flat on the floor or a step so that they are in a better position for pooing. Try to be calm and reassure them.

How paediatric osteopathy can help constipation

We have covered the key factors in this chapter that can contribute to constipation in babies and children. It is important to check these first. When treating a baby or child with constipation the focus should be on improving digestive clearance. Gentle muscular techniques to influence the breathing diaphragm which controls traction on the oesophagus. Cranial base muscular techniques are used to allow the vagus nerve to function effectively. I continue with lower digestive tract fascial tissue lengthening, to create colon clearance and establish regular peristalsis and finally, I ease the occiput-sacral tension by gentle techniques which balance the skeletal system.

Katie's story

Mum brought three-year-old Katie to see me at the clinic for constipation. Mum said Katie was born at 39 weeks after an uneventful labour lasting ten hours. There were no complications during labour, and both mum and baby were discharged after three days.

Mum breastfed Katie for four months and introduced a bottle after six weeks, with weaning from breast to bottle completed just after four months. When breastfed, Katie initially had two to four bowel motions a day. When weaned, Katie's bowel motions were every second day which is within normal.

Katie weaned onto solids at six months and enjoyed a wide range of food groups. It was at this time that Katie's mum noticed a change in her bowel habits. They slowed down to every three days and at times Katie was straining to go. The stools produced were toothpaste-like in consistency. Mum started to give Katie some orange juice or prune juice periodically and although this helped the straining pattern, bowel movements were still every three days.

Roll on to potty training at two and a half years and Katie's mum said that Katie found poos became difficult. Mum said that Katie got upset trying to go and became stressed by sitting on the potty. Katie would eventually go in a pull-up nappy. Her bowels were now opening every four days. Mum felt that Katie was holding and ignoring the urge to go. Mum took Katie to the doctor and the she prescribed Movicol daily to establish a more regular pattern. Mum said that Movicol helped Katie go more often, but she was still holding onto poos.

When I spoke to Mum about Katie and particularly asked about her daily hydration pattern, Mum said that Katie was poor at taking fluids. She was a very busy child and would take water and juice with meals only. I also asked about timing of using the toilet and Mum said they didn't have a schedule each day. I asked Mum to measure Katie's hydration for three days and to report back to me about her findings. I also suggested that she should look to schedule a toilet visit about an hour after meals and to continue with Movicol.

On cranial assessment I found a number of areas that required work, the lower abdominal area where bloating at the ascending and descending areas of the colon, tension in the lower ribcage and tension in the sub occipital muscle at the base of the skull. These areas were treated using gentle techniques to establish increased tissue flexibility.

When Mum returned a week later, she stated that having measured Katie's fluid intake for three days she said that the maximum Katie took was between 250–350mls per day. This was a significant finding as it should be at least 600mls per day. Dehydration affects bowel action. I advised Mum to increase Katie's fluid intake and continue to schedule time after meals for toileting. Treatment focused on the colon area again and easing tension in the lower ribcage to improve breathing diaphragm motion.

Next visit a week later was very positive. Katie had now a bowel motion each day, fluid intake was up and she was now using the toilet with confidence. Mum had spoken to her doctor and Movicol was now only to be used if bowels slowed again. I got a call from Mum three weeks later to say Katie was doing very well, bowels were opening daily and confidence using the toilet was established.

My main conclusions with this case were that fluid intake is a key area to check and stress-free toileting for the child is important. Treatment applied to the digestive system can stimulate activation of the bowel. Once a regular pattern is established it can remain once good habits are continued.

Symptom management chart

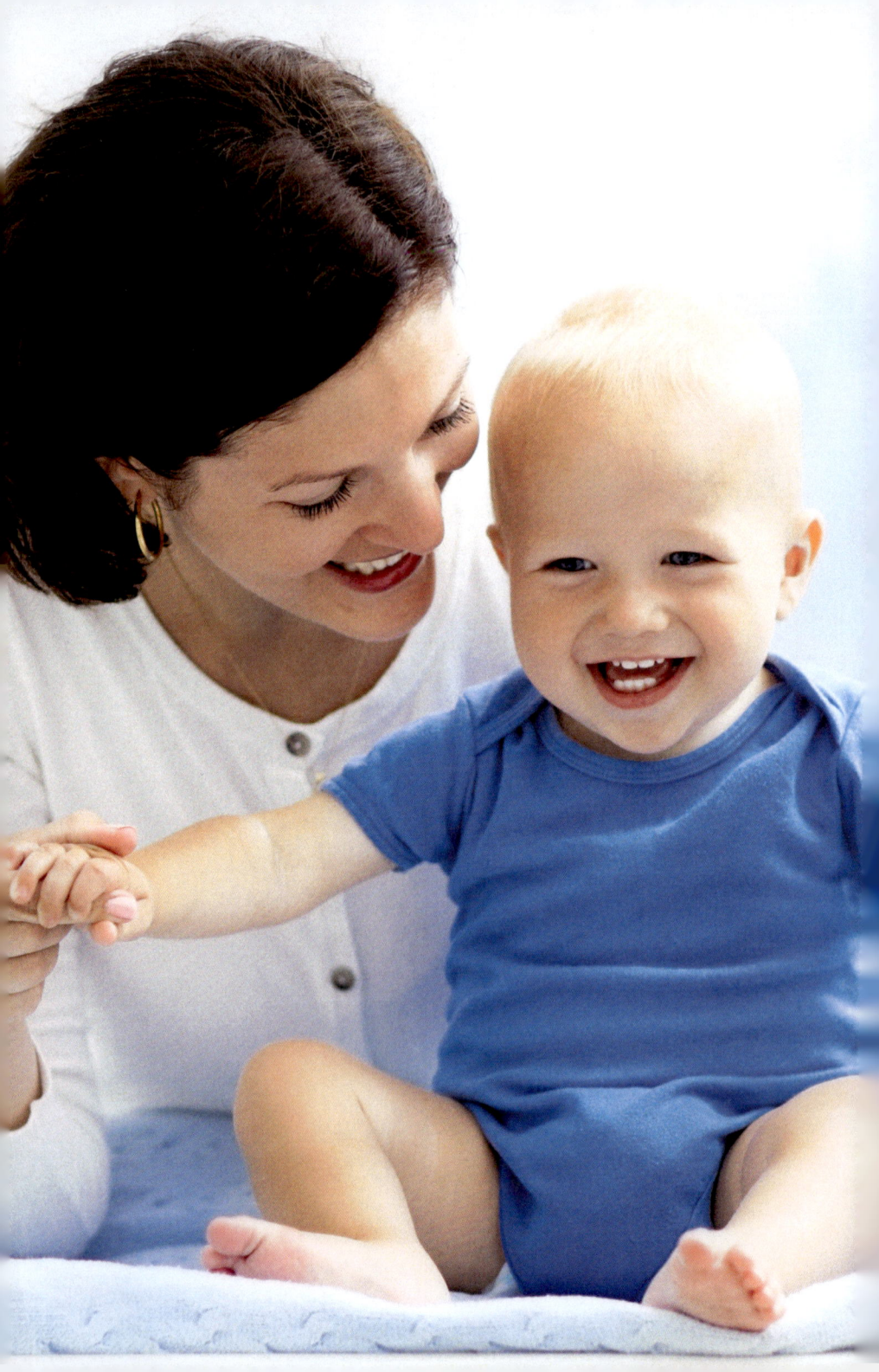

This chart allows you to monitor the changes in your baby after a management plan is put in place. It may be a change of formula, the addition of drops, medication or a dietary change. Whatever the plan, it's always a good idea to chart the next few days objectively. This will allow you to see any improvements that may otherwise be missed. A printable copy of this chart is available to download free from our website, www.corkchildrensclinic.com

How to use the symptom management chart

The chart looks at five main areas: crying, wind, sleep, bowels and feeding. By observing and grading these five areas you get a broad picture of how baby is over the full week. The chart allows you to be objective rather than subjective. So, when you are asked how baby is doing, you can give a more comprehensive picture of the week rather than saying "I think he's a little better, but he cried a lot last night so I'm not sure".

Towards the end of each day, think about the five key areas and grade each on your chart. If 9/10 is a baby who cries excessively for long periods of time and a 1/10 is a baby who only cries for a very short period after a feed/change, you get an idea of where your little one is. Similarly, with wind, a 10/10 would be a baby who is crying, pulling up his legs and in obvious distress for long periods with lower wind. A 1/10 would be a baby who burps easily and without upset after feeds.

Looking at each area separately builds up the picture, a bit like painting by numbers! It can be difficult to remain objective when it's your baby you are talking about, and you're tired and emotional. This chart will help you explain your concerns to your medical practitioner in a calm and informative way, and this in turn will lead to a more accurate diagnosis and review of the treatment plan.

To download a printable copy of this chart, go to:
www.corkchildrensclinic.com/freedownloads

Symptom Management Chart

List any changes to your baby's treatment plan below | Date:

1. | 2. | 3.

10/10 .... 5/10 .... 1/10
Very bad   Average   Very good

CRYING	10/10	9/10	8/10	7/10	6/10	5/10	4/10	3/10	2/10	1/10
Day 1										
Day 2										
Day 3										
Day 4										
Day 5										
Day 6										
Day 7										

WIND	10/10	9/10	8/10	7/10	6/10	5/10	4/10	3/10	2/10	1/10
Day 1										
Day 2										
Day 3										
Day 4										
Day 5										
Day 6										
Day 7										

SLEEP	10/10	9/10	8/10	7/10	6/10	5/10	4/10	3/10	2/10	1/10
Day 1										
Day 2										
Day 3										
Day 4										
Day 5										
Day 6										
Day 7										

BOWELS	10/10	9/10	8/10	7/10	6/10	5/10	4/10	3/10	2/10	1/10
Day 1										
Day 2										
Day 3										
Day 4										
Day 5										
Day 6										
Day 7										

FEEDING	10/10	9/10	8/10	7/10	6/10	5/10	4/10	3/10	2/10	1/10
Day 1										
Day 2										
Day 3										
Day 4										
Day 5										
Day 6										
Day 7										

SYMPTOM MANAGEMENT CHART

Symptom Management Chart

List any changes to your baby's treatment plan below	Date:
1.	
2.	3.

10/10 .... 5/10 .... 1/10

Very bad　　　　　　　Average　　　　　　　Very good

CRYING	10/10	9/10	8/10	7/10	6/10	5/10	4/10	3/10	2/10	1/10
Day 1										
Day 2										
Day 3										
Day 4										
Day 5										
Day 6										
Day 7										

WIND	10/10	9/10	8/10	7/10	6/10	5/10	4/10	3/10	2/10	1/10
Day 1										
Day 2										
Day 3										
Day 4										
Day 5										
Day 6										
Day 7										

SLEEP	10/10	9/10	8/10	7/10	6/10	5/10	4/10	3/10	2/10	1/10
Day 1										
Day 2										
Day 3										
Day 4										
Day 5										
Day 6										
Day 7										

BOWELS	10/10	9/10	8/10	7/10	6/10	5/10	4/10	3/10	2/10	1/10
Day 1										
Day 2										
Day 3										
Day 4										
Day 5										
Day 6										
Day 7										

FEEDING	10/10	9/10	8/10	7/10	6/10	5/10	4/10	3/10	2/10	1/10
Day 1										
Day 2										
Day 3										
Day 4										
Day 5										
Day 6										
Day 7										

NOTES

NOTES

NOTES

NOTES

For more information on Frank Kelleher,
paediatric osteopath see:
corkchildrensclinic.com

To download our *Symptom Checkers* and
our *Symptom Management Chart* see:
cherishedbabyandchild.com

For more information on osteopathy see:
osteopathy.org.uk
osteopathy.ie